ANATOMY
FOR YOGA

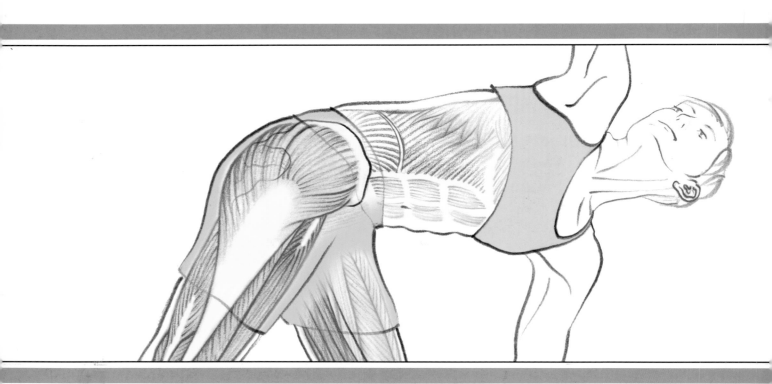

ANATOMY FOR YOGA

NICKY JENKINS AND LEIGH BRANDON

New York   Chicago   San Francisco   Lisbon   London
Madrid   Mexico City   Milan   New Delhi   San Juan
Seoul   Singapore   Sydney   Toronto

CONTENTS

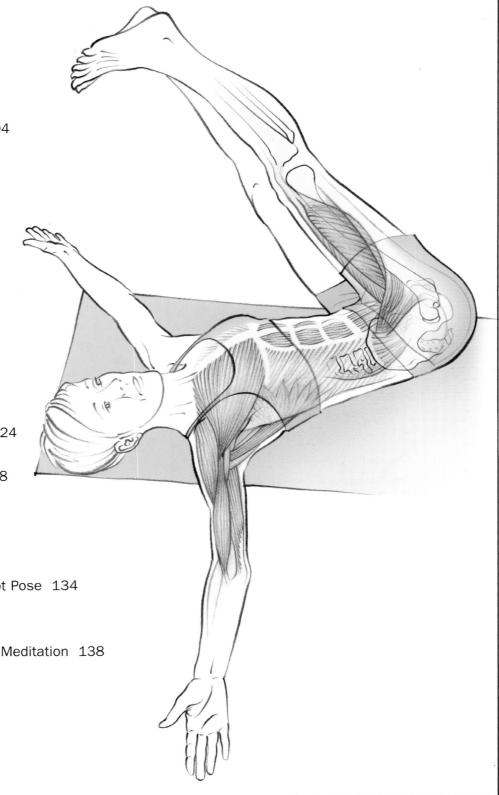

HOW TO USE THIS BOOK

Anatomy for Yoga is a visual and textual analysis of yoga poses, as well as a guide on how to perform the poses and how to safely and effectively improve your posture and your health. The book has two distinct parts: the first is a basic introduction to anatomical definitions, terminology, and an overview of posture, meditation, breath, and the chakras. Essentially, it helps demystify the language used in part two, making it easier to follow the instructions in that section. Part two contains four sections: section one covers kyphotic posture, section two covers lordotic posture, section three covers the flat-back posture, and section four covers the sway-back posture. Within each section are five subsections: the first covers the potential physical and emotional causes of the particular posture; the second focuses on the related chakra imbalances that may arise; the third section is the sequence of poses, where the individual poses are defined; and the fourth and fifth sections cover a breathing practice and a meditation practice. There is a "how to" guide for performing the poses in a sequence, as well as a visual and technical analysis of which muscles are being stretched and which muscles are active. The pose is depicted and technique tips are also included.

This book has been designed to help improve your posture and increase your vitality and health. Each pose has been specifically chosen to create balance within each postural type, so it is advisable to follow the sequence as it is shown. In order to understand which postural type you fall into (if any), have a trained professional assess your posture—this could be a physiotherapist, chiropractor, CHEK practitioner, or yoga teacher who has an understanding of postural imbalances. The four postures illustrated show the more advanced stages of postural deviation. Due to most people's day-to-day lives, many of us will suffer from some of these imbalances, but not to the same extreme. The sequences depicted in this book will assist in preventing further imbalances from occurring and help bring back muscular balance. When approaching the improvement of our posture, we must also look to enhance both our spiritual and emotional connection to our body. Through exploring the chakras and the possible emotional holding patterns, we can look into the root of our physical holding patterns and try to let them go. The breathing and meditation practices will help bring you to a place of inner stillness and understanding, bestowing upon you an inner strength that will manifest itself in confidence and the ability to "stand tall".

The adult human body has 639 muscles and 206 bones; this book illustrates many of the muscles involved in activation and stretching. Many smaller muscles, including the deep, small muscles of the spine and jaw and most muscles of the hands and feet, are not given specific attention.

Disclaimer: the poses have a small degree of risk of injury if done without adequate instruction and supervision. It is recommended that you begin with the easier modified poses and that you seek qualified instruction if you are a complete beginner. This book does not constitute medical advice, and the author and publisher cannot be held liable for any loss, injury, or inconvenience sustained by anyone using this book or the information contained within it.

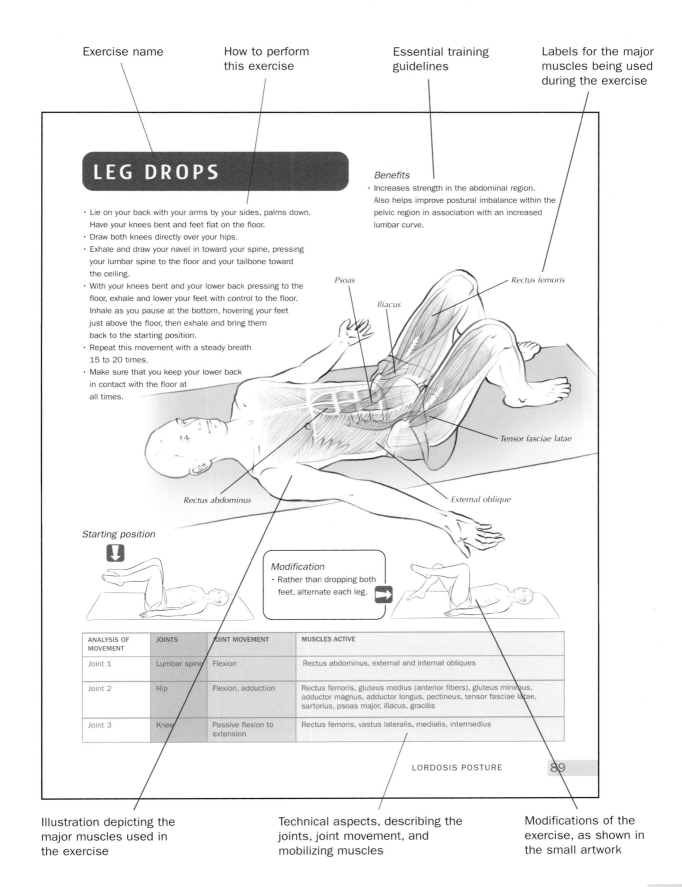

Exercise name

How to perform this exercise

Essential training guidelines

Labels for the major muscles being used during the exercise

LEG DROPS

- Lie on your back with your arms by your sides, palms down. Have your knees bent and feet flat on the floor.
- Draw both knees directly over your hips.
- Exhale and draw your navel in toward your spine, pressing your lumbar spine to the floor and your tailbone toward the ceiling.
- With your knees bent and your lower back pressing to the floor, exhale and lower your feet with control to the floor. Inhale as you pause at the bottom, hovering your feet just above the floor, then exhale and bring them back to the starting position.
- Repeat this movement with a steady breath 15 to 20 times.
- Make sure that you keep your lower back in contact with the floor at all times.

Benefits
- Increases strength in the abdominal region. Also helps improve postural imbalance within the pelvic region in association with an increased lumbar curve.

Psoas

Iliacus

Rectus femoris

Tensor fasciae latae

Rectus abdominus

External oblique

Starting position

Modification
- Rather than dropping both feet, alternate each leg.

ANALYSIS OF MOVEMENT	JOINTS	JOINT MOVEMENT	MUSCLES ACTIVE
Joint 1	Lumbar spine	Flexion	Rectus abdominus, external and internal obliques
Joint 2	Hip	Flexion, adduction	Rectus femoris, gluteus medius (anterior fibers), gluteus minimus, adductor magnus, adductor longus, pectineus, tensor fasciae latae, sartorius, psoas major, iliacus, gracilis
Joint 3	Knee	Passive flexion to extension	Rectus femoris, vastus lateralis, medialis, intermedius

LORDOSIS POSTURE 89

Illustration depicting the major muscles used in the exercise

Technical aspects, describing the joints, joint movement, and mobilizing muscles

Modifications of the exercise, as shown in the small artwork

PART 1. OVERVIEW OF ANATOMY

ANATOMICAL DEFINITIONS AND TERMINOLOGY

Anatomy has its own language, and, while technical, it has a basis in logic, originating from the Latin and Greek root words that make it easier to learn and understand the names of muscles, bones, and other body parts. Whether you're a yoga instructor or student, using the correct terminology enables you to interact with other professionals and professional materials.

Like most medical terms, anatomical terms are made up of small word parts, known as combining forms, that fit together to make the full term. These "combining forms" comprise roots, prefixes, and suffixes. Knowing the different word parts allows you to unravel the word. Most anatomical terms contain only two parts: either a prefix and root or a root and suffix.

For example, if you take the terms subscapular and suprascapular, the root is "scapula," commonly known as the shoulder blade. "Supra" means "above" so "suprascapula" means something above the shoulder blade and "sub" means "below," indicating, in this instance, something below the shoulder blade.

Common prefixes, suffixes, and roots of anatomical terms

Word root	Meaning	Example	Definition
abdomin	pertaining to the abdomen	abdominal muscle	major muscle group of the abdominal region
acro	extremity	acromion	protruding feature on the scapula bone
articul	pertaining to the joint	articular surface	joint surface
brachi	pertaining to the arm	brachialis	arm muscle
cerv	pertaining to the neck	cervical vertebrae	the neck region of the spine
crani	skull	cranium	bones forming the skull
glute	buttock	gluteus maximus	buttock muscle
lig	to tie, to bind	ligament	joins bone to bone
pector	chest region	pectoralis major	chest muscle
Word parts used as prefixes			
ab-	away from, from, off	abduction	movement away from the midline
ad-	increase, adherence, toward	adduction	movement toward the midline
ante-, antero-	before, in front	anterior	front aspect of the body
bi-	two, double	biceps brachii	two-headed arm muscle
circum-	around	circumduction	circular movement of a limb
cleido-	the clavicle	sternocleiomastoid	muscle, inserts into clavicle
con-	with, together	concentric contraction	contraction in which muscle attachments move together

Word parts used as prefixes (continued)

Word root	Meaning	Example	Definition
costo-	rib	costal cartilage	rib cartilage
cune-	wedge	cuneiform	wedge-shaped foot bone
de-	down from	depression	downward movement of the shoulder blades
dors-	back	dorsiflexion	movement of the top side of the foot toward the shin
ec-	away from	eccentric contractions	contraction in which muscle attachments move apart
epi-	upon	epicondyle	feature of a bone, located above a condyle
fasci-	band	tensor fasciae latae	small, bandlike muscle of the hip
flex-	bend	flexion	movement closing the angle of a joint
infra-	below, beneath	infraspinatus	muscle situated below the spine of the scapula
meta-	after, behind	metatarsals	bones of the foot, distal to the tarsals
post-	after, behind	posterior	rear aspect of the body
pron-	bent forward	prone position	lying face-down
proximo-	nearest	proximal	nearest the root of a limb
quadr-	four	quadriceps	four-part muscle group on the anterior thigh
re-	back, again	retraction	pulling of the shoulder blades toward the midline
serrat-	saw	serratus anterior	muscle with a sawlike edge
sub-	beneath, inferior	subscapularis	muscle beneath the scapula
super-, supra-	over, above, excessive	supraspinatus	muscle above the spine of the scapula
		superior	toward the head
thoraco-	chest, thorax	thoracic vertebrae	in the region of the thorax
trans-	across	transverse abdominus	muscle crossing the abdomen
tri-	three	triceps brachii	three-headed muscle of the upper arm
tuber-	swelling	tubercle	small, rounded projection on a bone

Word parts used as suffixes

Word root	Meaning	Example	Definition
-al, ac	pertaining to	iliac crest	pertaining to the ilium
-cep	head	biceps brachii	two-headed arm muscle
-ic	pertaining to	thoracic vertebrae	pertaining to the thorax
-oid	like, in the shape of	rhomboid	upper back muscle, in the shape of a rhomboid
-phragm	partition	diaphragm	muscle separating the thorax and abdomen

The human body can be viewed as an integration of approximately 12 distinct systems that continuously interact to control a multitude of complex functions. These systems are a coordinated assembly of organs, each with specific capabilities, whose tissue structures suit a similar purpose and function.

This book illustrates and analyzes the systems that control movement and posture, namely the muscular and skeletal systems, often referred to jointly as the musculoskeletal system.

The other systems are the cardiovascular, lymphatic, nervous, endocrine, integumentary, respiratory, digestive, urinary, immune, and reproductive systems.

The muscular system

The muscular system facilitates movement, maintenance of posture, and the production of heat and energy. It is made up of three types of muscle tissues: cardiac, smooth, and striated.

Cardiac muscle forms the walls in the heart, while smooth muscle tissue is found in the walls of internal organs, such as the stomach and blood vessels. Both are activated involuntarily via the autonomic nervous system and hormonal action.

Striated muscle makes up the bulk of the muscles as we commonly know them. The skeletal system includes the tendons that attach muscle to bone, as well as the connective tissue that surrounds the muscle tissue, called fascia.

A human male weighing 154 lbs. (70 kg) has approximately 55–77 lbs. (25–35 kg) of skeletal tissue.

Muscle attachments

Muscles attach to bone via tendons. The attachment points are referred to as the origin and the insertion.

The origin is the point of attachment that is proximal (closest to the root of a limb) or closest to the midline, or center of the body. It is usually the least movable point, acting as the anchor in muscle contraction.

The insertion is the point of attachment that is distal (farthest from the root of a limb) or farthest from the midline, or center of the body. The insertion is usually the most movable part, and can be drawn toward the origin.

Knowing the origin and insertion of a muscle, which joint or joints the muscle crosses, and what movement is caused at that joint or joints, is a key element of exercise analysis.

There are typical features on all bones that act as convenient attachment points for the muscles. A description of typical bone features is given in the table opposite.

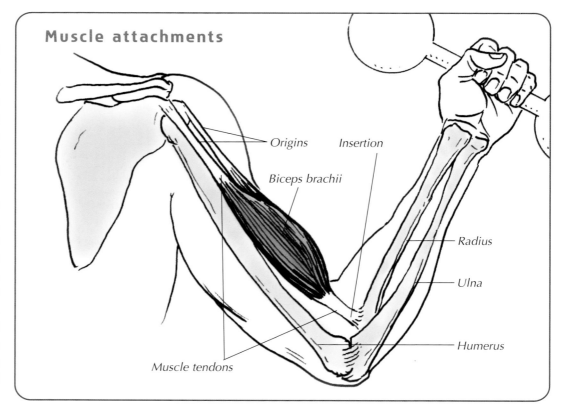

Muscle attachments

Origins

Insertion

Biceps brachii

Radius

Ulna

Humerus

Muscle tendons

Typical features on a bone

Feature	Description	Examples
Condyle	Large, rounded projection at a joint that usually articulates with another bone	Medial and lateral condyle of the femur Lateral condyle of the tibia
Epicondyle	Projection located above the condyle	Medial or lateral epicondyle of the humerus
Facet	Small, flat joint surfaces	Facet joints of the vertebrae
Head	Significant, rounded projection at the proximal end of a bone, usually forming a joint	Head of the humerus
Crest	Ridgelike, narrow projection	Iliac crest of the pelvis
Line, Linea	Lesser significant ridge, running along a bone	Linea aspera of the femur
Process	Any significant projection	Coracoid and acromion process of the scapula Olecranon process of the ulna at the elbow joint
Spine, Spinous process	Significant, slender projection away from the surface of the bone	Spinous processes of the vertebrae Spine of the scapula
Suture	Joint line between two bones forming a fixed or semifixed joint	Sutures that join the bones of the skull
Trochanter	Very large projection	Greater trochanter of the femur
Tubercle	Small, rounded projection	Greater tubercles of the humerus
Tuberosity	Large, rounded or roughened projection	Ischial tuberosities on the pelvis
Foramen	Rounded hole or opening in a bone	The vertebral foramen running down the length of the spine, in which the spinal cord is housed
Fossa	Hollow, shallow, or flattened surface on a bone	Supraspinous and infraspinous fossa on the scapula

The word "skeleton" originates from a Greek word meaning "dried up." Infants are born with about 350 bones, many of which fuse as they grow, forming single bones, resulting in the 206 bones of an adult.

The muscular system

Anterior view

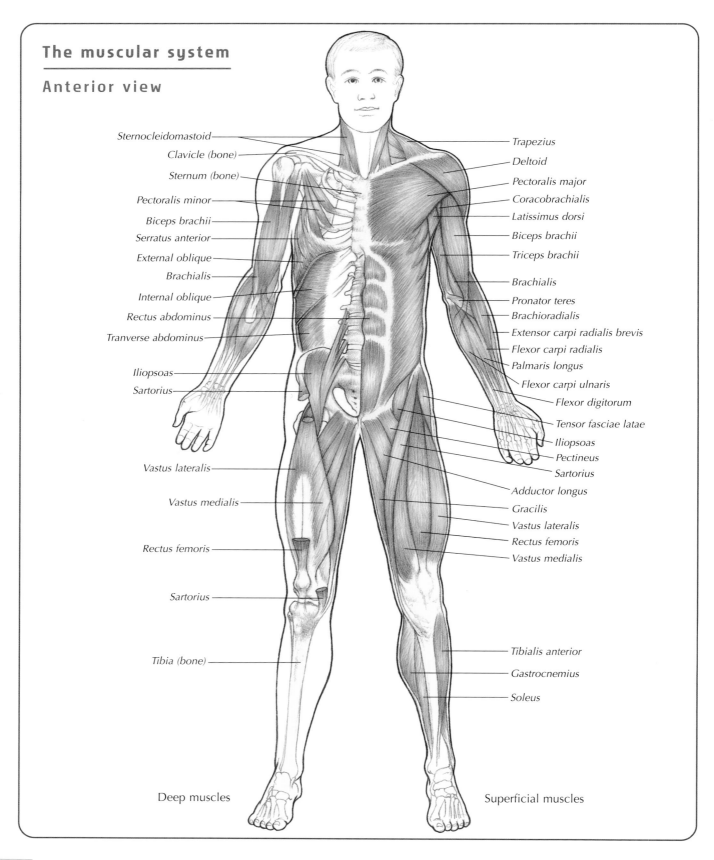

Sternocleidomastoid
Clavicle (bone)
Sternum (bone)
Pectoralis minor
Biceps brachii
Serratus anterior
External oblique
Brachialis
Internal oblique
Rectus abdominus
Tranverse abdominus
Iliopsoas
Sartorius
Vastus lateralis
Vastus medialis
Rectus femoris
Sartorius
Tibia (bone)

Trapezius
Deltoid
Pectoralis major
Coracobrachialis
Latissimus dorsi
Biceps brachii
Triceps brachii
Brachialis
Pronator teres
Brachioradialis
Extensor carpi radialis brevis
Flexor carpi radialis
Palmaris longus
Flexor carpi ulnaris
Flexor digitorum
Tensor fasciae latae
Iliopsoas
Pectineus
Sartorius
Adductor longus
Gracilis
Vastus lateralis
Rectus femoris
Vastus medialis
Tibialis anterior
Gastrocnemius
Soleus

Deep muscles

Superficial muscles

The muscular system

Posterior view

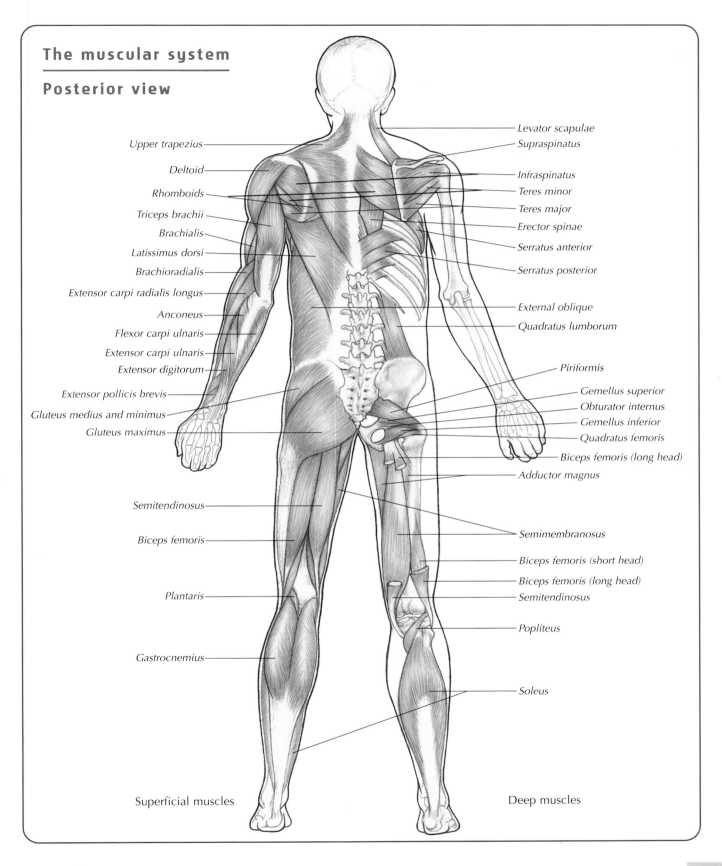

Upper trapezius

Deltoid

Rhomboids

Triceps brachii

Brachialis

Latissimus dorsi

Brachioradialis

Extensor carpi radialis longus

Anconeus

Flexor carpi ulnaris

Extensor carpi ulnaris

Extensor digitorum

Extensor pollicis brevis

Gluteus medius and minimus

Gluteus maximus

Semitendinosus

Biceps femoris

Plantaris

Gastrocnemius

Levator scapulae

Supraspinatus

Infraspinatus

Teres minor

Teres major

Erector spinae

Serratus anterior

Serratus posterior

External oblique

Quadratus lumborum

Piriformis

Gemellus superior

Obturator internus

Gemellus inferior

Quadratus femoris

Biceps femoris (long head)

Adductor magnus

Semimembranosus

Biceps femoris (short head)

Biceps femoris (long head)

Semitendinosus

Popliteus

Soleus

Superficial muscles

Deep muscles

The skeletal system

This consists of bones, ligaments (which join bone to bone), and joints. Joints are referred to as articulations and are sometimes classified as a separate system, called the articular system.

Aside from facilitating movement, the primary functions of the skeletal system include supporting the muscles, protecting the soft tissues and internal organs, storing surplus minerals, and forming red blood cells in the bone marrow of the long bones.

Integrated systems

The body's systems are completely and intricately interdependent. In order for movement to take place, for example, the respiratory system brings in oxygen and the digestive system breaks down our food into essential nutrients. The cardiovascular system then carries the oxygen and nutrients to the working muscles via the blood to facilitate the energy reactions that result in physical work being done.

The lymphatic and circulatory systems help carry away the waste products of these energy reactions, which are later converted and/or excreted by the digestive and urinary systems. The nervous system interacts with the muscles to facilitate the contraction and relaxation of the muscle tissue. The articular system of joints allows the levers of the body to move.

The femur (thighbone) is about one fourth of a person's height. It is also the largest, heaviest, and strongest bone in the body. The shortest bone, the stapes (or stirrup) bone in the ear, is only about 0.1 in. (2.5 mm) long. An adult's skeleton weighs about 20 lbs. (9 kg).

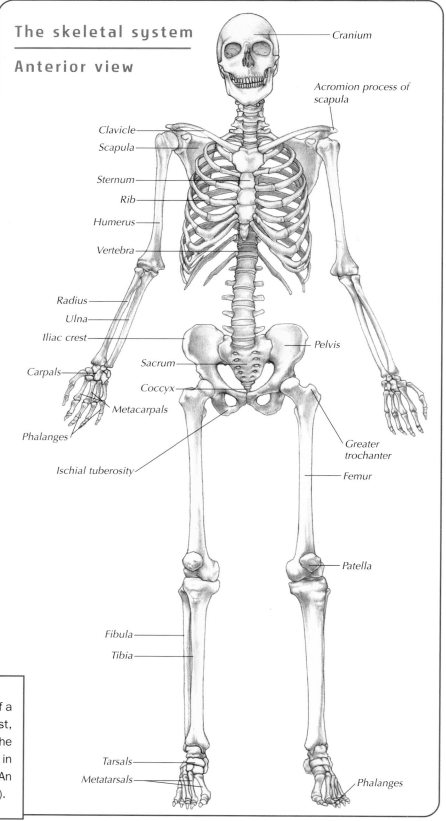

The skeletal system

Anterior view

Cranium
Acromion process of scapula
Clavicle
Scapula
Sternum
Rib
Humerus
Vertebra
Radius
Ulna
Iliac crest
Carpals
Sacrum
Coccyx
Metacarpals
Phalanges
Ischial tuberosity
Pelvis
Greater trochanter
Femur
Patella
Fibula
Tibia
Tarsals
Metatarsals
Phalanges

BODY PLANES AND REGIONS

When learning anatomy and analyzing movement, we refer to a standard reference position of the human body, known as the anatomical position (see illustration below). All movements and locations of anatomical structures are named as if the person were standing in this position.

Regional anatomy

This book is a technical labeling guide to the different superficial parts of the body. In anatomical language, common names such as "head" are replaced with anatomical terms derived from Latin, such as "cranial" or "cranium."

Within the different body regions there are subregions. For example, within the cranial region are the frontal, occipital, parietal, and temporal subregions.

Anatomical planes

The body can be divided into three imaginary planes of reference, each one perpendicular to the other.

The sagittal plane passes through the body from front to back, dividing it into a right half and a left half. The midline of the body is called the median. If the body is divided in the sagittal plane, directly through its median, this is known as the median sagittal plane. The coronal (frontal plane) passes through the body from top to bottom, dividing it into front and back sections.

The transverse (horizontal) plane passes through the middle of the body at right angles, dividing it into a top and a bottom section.

An anatomical crosssection of the internal structures of the body can be viewed in any one of these planes, which are also described as "planes of motion," as the joint movements are defined in relation to one of the three planes. Understanding into which plane an anatomical crosssection is divided will help you know what you are looking at and from which viewpoint.

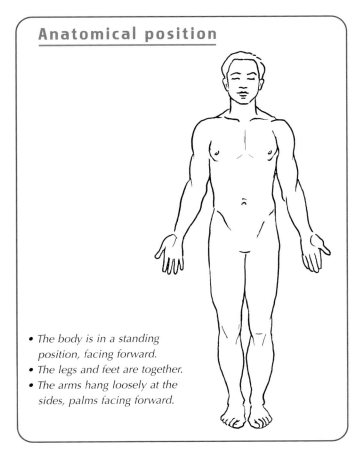

Anatomical position

- The body is in a standing position, facing forward.
- The legs and feet are together.
- The arms hang loosely at the sides, palms facing forward.

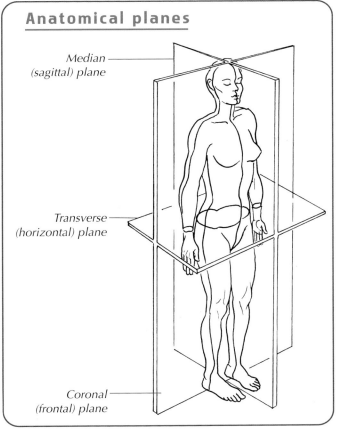

Anatomical planes

Median (sagittal) plane

Transverse (horizontal) plane

Coronal (frontal) plane

ANATOMICAL TERMS

There are standard anatomical terms that describe the position or direction of one structure of the body and its relationship to other structures or parts of the body.

The human body is a complex, three-dimensional structure. Knowing the proper anatomical terms of position and direction will help you compare one point on the body with another and understand where it is situated in relation to other anatomical features.

These terms are standard, no matter whether the person is standing, seated, or lying down, and are named as if the person were standing in the anatomical position (see previous page). The terms of direction should not be confused with joint movements (see pages 17–20).

Anatomical terms of position and direction

Position	Definition	Example of usage
Anterior	Toward the front, pertaining to the front	The pectoral muscles are found on the anterior aspect of the body
Posterior	Toward the back, pertaining to the back	The calf muscles are situated on the posterior surface of the lower leg
Superior	Above another structure, toward the head	The knee is superior to the ankle
Inferior	Below another structure, toward the feet	The hip is inferior to the shoulder
Lateral	Away from the midline, on or toward the outside	The radial bone is lateral to the ulna
Medial	Toward the midline, pertaining to the middle or center	The tibial bone is medial to the fibula
Proximal	Closest to the trunk or root of a limb; sometimes used to refer to the origin of a muscle	The shoulder joint is proximal to the elbow
Distal	Situated away from the midline or center of the body or root of a limb; sometimes used to refer to a point away from the origin of a muscle	The knee joint is distal to the hip
Superficial	Closer to the surface of the body, more toward the surface of the body than another structure	The rectus abdominus is the most superficial muscle of the abdominal wall
Deep	Farther from the surface, relatively deeper into the body than another structure	The transverse abdominus is the deepest muscle of the abdominal wall
Prone	Lying face-down	A prone cobra exercise is performed from a lying starting position
Supine	Lying on the back, face upward	A bench-press exercise is performed from a supine position

JOINT MOVEMENTS

Knowing and understanding movement (which joint is moving and how it moves) is essential in order to analyze a complex exercise. This book has done the task of joint identification for you, and understanding this section will help improve your exercise analysis.

Types of joints

Some joints are fixed or semifixed, allowing little or no movement. For instance, the bones of the skull connect in structures known as sutures to form fixed joints; but where the spine joins the pelvis, the sacroiliac ("sacro" from sacrum and "iliac" pertaining to the pelvic crest) joint is semifixed and allows minimal movement.

A third category called synovial joints are free-moving and move in different ways determined by their particular shape, size, and structure. Synovial joints are the most common joints in the body. They are categorized by a joint capsule that surrounds the articulation, the inner membrane of which secretes lubricating synovial fluid, stimulated by movement. Typical synovial joints include the shoulder, knee, hip, ankle, joints of the feet and hands, and the vertebral joints.

Joint action

When performing an activity such as yoga, walking, or running, the combination of nerve stimulation and muscular contraction facilitates the movement that occurs at the synovial joints.

When doing a "down dog," for example (see page 50), the body weight rises away from the floor because the angle of the ankle, knee, and hip joints decreases due to the muscles acting across the joints contracting and causing the joints to flex.

Joint movement pointers

Most joint movements have common names that apply to most major joints, but there are some movements that occur at only one specific joint.

The common joint movements occur in similar anatomical planes of motion. For example, shoulder, hip, and knee flexion all occur in the sagittal plane (see page 15). This makes it logical and easier to learn about both joint movements and movement analysis.

In the table below, common movements are listed first, followed by specific movements that only occur at one joint.

Strictly speaking, it is incorrect to name only the movement and a limb or body part. For example, "leg extension" does not clarify if this happens at the knee, hip, or ankle. Get into the habit of always pairing the movement with the joint that is moved. For example, elbow flexion, hip extension, spinal rotation, and scapular elevation. (Possibly the only exception to this is when referring to trunk movements, when all the joints of the spine combine to create movement of the whole body part.)

Movements generally occur in pairs. For every movement, there must be a return movement to the starting position. Typical pairs are flexion and extension, abduction and adduction, internal rotation and external rotation, protraction and retraction, and elevation and depression.

Remember that all movements are named as if the person were standing in the anatomical position (see page 15). So "elbow flexion" is the same regardless of whether you are standing, seated, or lying down (supine).

Major joint movements

General movements	Plane	Description
Abduction	Coronal	Movement away from the midline
Adduction	Coronal	Movement toward the midline
Flexion	Sagittal	Decreasing the angle between two structures
Extension	Sagittal	Increasing the angle between two structures
Medial rotation (internal rotation)	Transverse	Turning around the vertical axis of a bone toward the midline

Lateral rotation (external rotation)	Transverse	Turning around the vertical axis of a bone away from the midline
Circumduction	All planes	Complete circular movement at shoulder or hip joints

Specific movements		

1. Ankle movements		
Plantarflexion	Sagittal	Moving the toes downward
Dorsiflexion	Sagittal	Moving the foot toward the shin

2. Forearm movements (the radioulnar joint)		
Pronation	Transverse	Rotating the hand and wrist medially from the elbow
Supination	Transverse	Rotating the hand and wrist laterally from the elbow

3. Scapula movements		
Depression	Coronal	Movement of the scapulae inferiorly, e.g. squeezing the scapulae downward
Elevation	Coronal	Movement of the scapulae superiorly, e.g. hunching the scapulae upward
Abduction (protraction)	Transverse	Movement of the scapulae away from the spine
Adduction (retraction)	Transverse	Movement of the scapulae toward the spine
Downward rotation	Coronal	Scapulae rotates downward, in the return from upward rotation
Upward rotation	Coronal	Scapulae rotate upward. The inferior angle of the scapula moves upward and laterally

4. Shoulder movements		
Horizontal abduction/extension	Transverse	Movement of the humerus across the body, away from the midline
Horizontal adduction/flexion	Transverse	Movement of the humerus across the body, toward the midline

5. Spine/trunk movements		
Lateral flexion	Coronal	Movement of the trunk away from the midline
	Coronal	Return of the trunk toward the midline in the coronal plane

6. Wrist movements		
Ulnar deviation	Coronal	Movement of the hand toward the midline from the anatomical position
Radial deviation	Coronal	Movement of the hand away from the midline from the anatomical position

Joint movements

The knee joint is the largest, the hip joint is the strongest, and the shoulder is potentially the most unstable joint in the body.

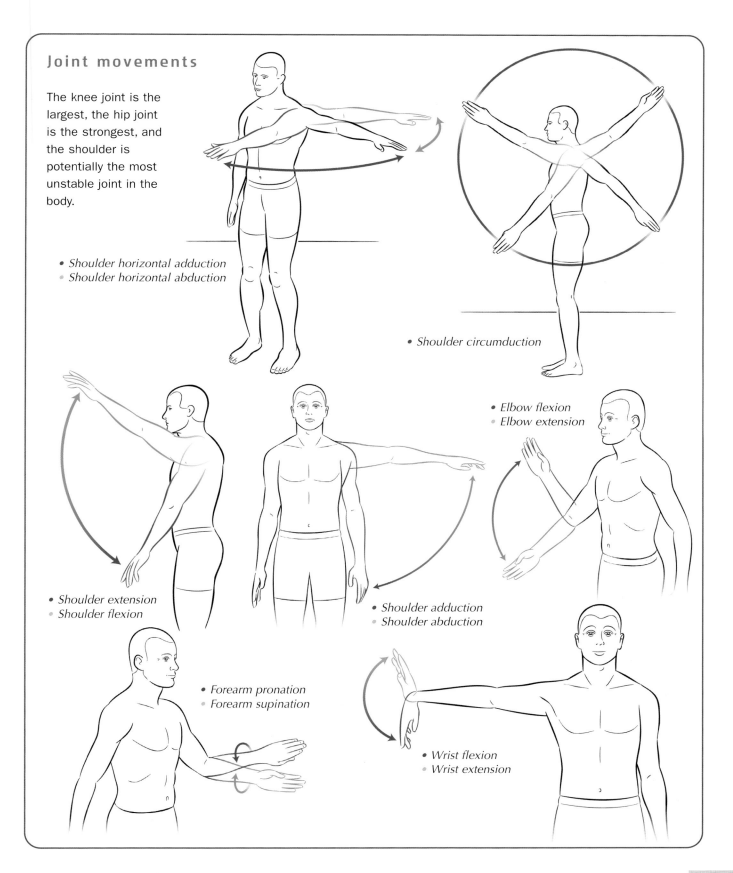

- *Shoulder horizontal adduction*
- *Shoulder horizontal abduction*

- *Shoulder circumduction*

- *Shoulder extension*
- *Shoulder flexion*

- *Shoulder adduction*
- *Shoulder abduction*

- *Elbow flexion*
- *Elbow extension*

- *Forearm pronation*
- *Forearm supination*

- *Wrist flexion*
- *Wrist extension*

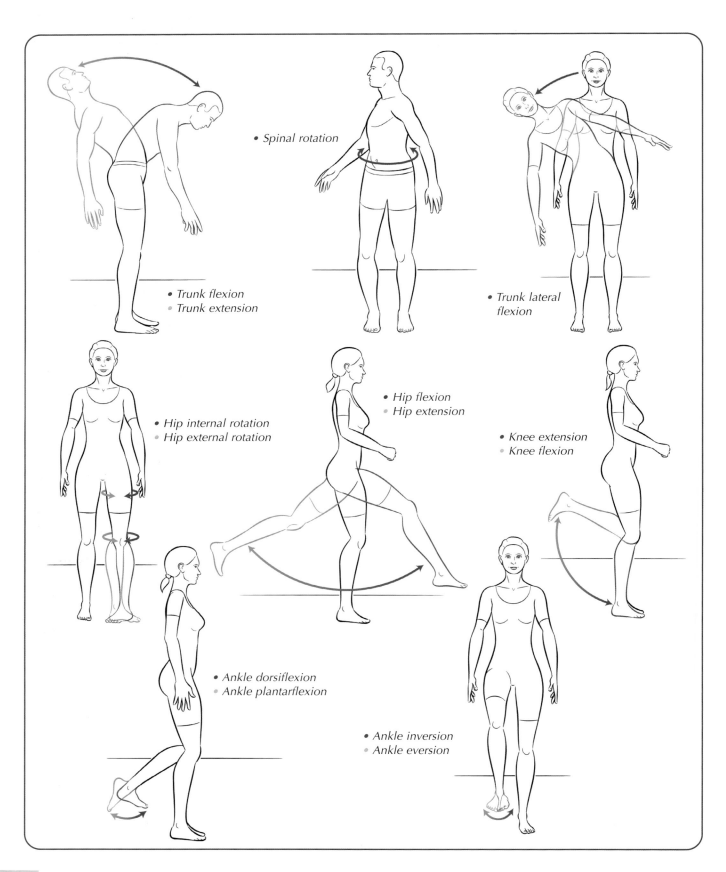

- *Spinal rotation*

- *Trunk flexion*
- *Trunk extension*

- *Trunk lateral flexion*

- *Hip internal rotation*
- *Hip external rotation*

- *Hip flexion*
- *Hip extension*

- *Knee extension*
- *Knee flexion*

- *Ankle dorsiflexion*
- *Ankle plantarflexion*

- *Ankle inversion*
- *Ankle eversion*

OVERVIEW OF ANATOMY

POSTURE AND MUSCLE BALANCE

Posture has become something of a buzz word in recent years. However, the understanding, importance, and methods of correcting posture are often misunderstood.

There are many definitions of posture. They include:

"The position from which all movement begins and ends." (Joel E. Goldthwaite)

"The position of the limbs or carriage of the body as a whole." (Stedman's Medical Dictionary)

"The position from which the musculoskeletal system functions most efficiently." (Moshe Feldenkrais)

In addition to these definitions, there are also two main categories of posture: static and dynamic.

Static posture

Static posture may be defined as "the position of the body at rest, sitting, standing, or lying" (P. Chek, *Golf Biomechanics Manual*). This means that if you have poor posture before you are moving, you will have poor posture while moving. Therefore, poor static posture will be expressed in your movements.

Dynamic posture

Dynamic posture may be defined as "the ability to maintain an optimal instantaneous axis of rotation of any/all working joints in any time/space relationship—regardless of body position or speed of movement" (P. Chek, *Golf Biomechanics Certification Course Manual*).

As a simple analogy, you can think of your spine as an axis of rotation (like a crankshaft) and your arms as a means by which motion at the axis is expressed (like the connecting rod). If your spinal axis is faulty and expresses the exaggerated curvatures that go hand in hand with poor posture, your capacity to rotate efficiently will be significantly reduced. If your spinal axis is correctly aligned, you are far more efficient and are likely to move and perform to your full potential.

Optimal posture is maintained when muscles surrounding a joint or joints are in balance. Good "muscle balance" simply means that the muscles are at their optimal or normal length and tension. A muscle imbalance is when a muscle on one side of a joint is tight and its opposing muscle (antagonist) is long and potentially weak. This causes the joint to lose its optimal axis of rotation, which can lead to excessive wear and tear on the joint and increase the likelihood of injury during physical activity.

Posture and alignment

The gravitational pull that is exerted on the body acts through the body in a straight line toward the center of the earth.

In a standing position, neutral alignment occurs when body landmarks, such as the ankles, knees, hips, shoulders, and ears, are in line with the pull of gravity. The body also requires balance from front to back and side to side, allowing it to maintain its position against gravity with minimal effort. The more the body is out of alignment, the more

energy it uses to resist the gravitational pull. For most people, poor posture will not increase the likelihood of injury, but it will waste vital energy and could make you feel tired and unable to participate in all the things you enjoy doing.

In neutral alignment, the pelvis is in a neutral position with the pubic ramus and the anterior superior iliac crest vertically aligned (see overleaf). In this position, if the pelvis were a bucket of water, no water would spill out. With an anterior pelvic tilt, the water would pour out the front, and a posterior pelvic tilt would cause the water to pour out the back.

As we exercise and move the body in different positions, for example, when performing sun salutations (see page 48), gravity continues to affect the body, the critical points of balance shift, and we are required to work harder to maintain balance and alignment. Despite the fact that balance is shifting when peforming yoga, in most instances it is still important to maintain a neutral spine. "Neutral spine" in the instance of performing a "down dog" (see page 50) would require the maintenance of a straight line through the ear, shoulder, and pelvis, but not necessarily in a vertical line.

Poor postural control and alignment affect your quality of movement and the safety and effectiveness of any exercise, as postural compensation is likely to occur. This means that the joints used, joint actions, range of movement, and involvement of the various stabilizing and mobilizing muscles will change from the ideal. This increases the likelihood of injury.

Stabilizers and mobilizers

One common classification of muscles is whether they are performing a stabilizing or mobilizing function.

A mobilizer muscle is primarily responsible for creating movement across joints, for example, the iliospaos while moving into the "down dog" position (see page 50).

Stabilizers are muscles whose prime purpose in the body or in a given movement is to maintain the stability and alignment of the rest of the body, so that effective movement can be performed by the mobilizing muscles. For example, during the holding of a yogic pose, all the muscles perform a stabilizing role. Certain muscles, by virtue of their position, shape, angle, and muscle fiber type, are more suited to work as stabilizers than as mobilizers. Stablizing muscles tend to be deep in the joint and have lots of endurance but can't produce much power. Mobilizer muscles tend to be more superficial, have little endurance, but can produce a lot of power.

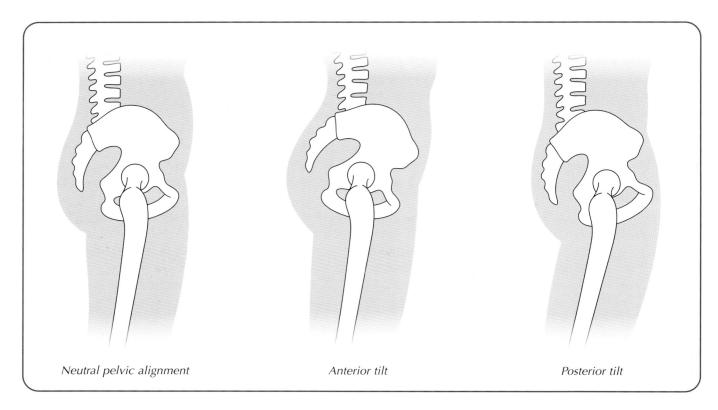

Neutral pelvic alignment   Anterior tilt   Posterior tilt

THE SPINE

The human spine is made up of 33 bones in five distinct regions. The five regions are the cervical, thoracic, lumbar, sacral, and coccygeal (coccyx).

Each vertebra has a vertebral body, a spinous process, and two transverse processes. Processes are bony protrusions that serve as attachment sites for muscles and ligaments. The spinous process protrudes directly posterior to the vertebral body, and the transverse processes protrude each side of the vertebral body superiorly just behind the midline. The angle of the processes in the sagittal plane vary all along the spine.

The spinal joints are called zygopophyseal joints, or facet joints. Each vertebra (except for the first two vertebrae) has a superior facet that articulates with the inferior facet on the vertebra above it. These joints limit the amount of side flexion, extension, and rotation.

Each vertebra is named according to the region in which it is located within the spine and in numerical order superiorly to inferiorly. For instance, the seven cervical vertebrae are named C1, C2, C3, C4, C5, C6, and C7. The first cervical vertebra is also known as the "atlas" and the second cervical vertebra is known as the "axis." The 12 thoracic vertebrae are listed T1–T12, the lumbar vertebrae are listed L1–L5, and the sacral vertebrae (even though they are fused) are listed S1–S5.

The vertebrae are separated by intervertebral disks made from fibrocartilage. The disks comprise of a nucleus polposus and an annulus fibrosis.

The nucleus polposus is a soft gel-like material in the center of the disk. The annulus fibrosis is less pliable and surrounds the nucleus polposis in concentric layers. The disks provide shock absorption, limit excessive movement of joints, and, according to Serge Gracovetsky (in *Collagen and the Second Law of Thermodynamics*), transfer kinetic energy during human gait, which enables efficiency of movement.

Movement is possible in all three planes of motion in the vertebrae. The only exceptions are the sacral and coccygeal regions, which are fused. The sacrum can, however, flex on the ilium of the pelvis by approximately four degrees (N. Bogduk, *Clinical Anatomy of the Lumbar Spine and Sacrum*).

The normal positions of the spinal curves in the anatomical position are as follows:

- Cervical: 30–35 degrees anteriorly
- Thoracic: 30–35 degrees posteriorly
- Lumbar: 30–35 degrees anteriorly

An anterior curvature of the spine is known as a lordosis. A posterior curvature of the spine is known as a kyphosis. A lateral curvature of the spine is known as a scoliosis. An increase in the lordotic curvature beyond the normal range is called hyperlordotic posture, and a decrease in curvature is known as a hypolordotic posture. The same use of the words "hyper" and "hypo" can be used when describing abnormal kyphotic postures.

The position of the cervical spine is crucial, as it forms the foundation for the head, where all the vital survival reflex mechanisms reside, such as breathing, chewing, vision, hearing, and balance.

In the anatomical position, the head should sit on the cervical spine with the eyes, ears, and jaw all level with the horizon, and the head should naturally sit on the cervical spine without any rotation or side flexion. When the head sits off this central position, it suggests an unnatural rotation or "subluxation" at the level of C1 on the occiput (base of the skull). This is known as an "atlas subluxation."

An atlas subluxation can be caused by trauma to the body or an attempt to realign the head level with the horizon due to an existing imbalance to one of the survival reflex mechanisms.

The position of the cervical spine is very dependant on the position of the thoracic spine. If the thoracic spine is in a hyperkyphotic position, the cervical spine has to compensate to keep the eyes level with the horizon. The cervical spine compensates by extending, which shortens the cervical extensors and lengthens and potentially weakens the cervical flexors.

The thoracic and lumbar spine positions are closely related, and their effects on each other are discussed in the next section.

According to Gracovetsky (*Collagen and the Second Law of Thermodynamics*), the human spine has developed through evolution from the reptile's spine. The reptile was the first creature to walk on land, and its spine flexes laterally like a fish's. The mammal's spine then used flexion and extension to ambulate more quickly than the reptile. The combination of flexion, extension, and lateral flexion also created rotation, which is used by primates and humans for ambulation (movement).

In a human spine, the whole of the cervical spine and the top half of the thoracic spine rotate and side-flex to the same side, e.g. when the neck side-bends to the right, there is a natural degree of right rotation, too.

However, in the lower half of the thoracic spine and the whole of the lumbar spine it is different. When the lumbar spine side-bends to the right, there is a natural rotation to the left and vice versa.

This is particularly important for professionals to understand when prescribing exercises for clients with back injuries.

Whenever someone has less than optimal posture or muscle imbalance, the following negative effects take place:

- Joints are unable to move through their instantaneous optimal axis of rotation.
- Therefore, entrapment of tendons, ligaments, blood vessels, and nerves can occur.
- This can lead to tendon tears (strains), ligament tears (sprains), nerve entrapment, and restriction of blood flow to tissues. It can also lead to excessive wear of the cartilage in joints.
- Joints can also be restricted from moving through their full range of motion. This will increase the likelihood of injury to muscles, tendons, and ligaments, especially during high-intensity exercise that require a wide range of motion.

Reciprocal inhibition

This occurs when a muscle tightens on one side of the joint. The opposing muscle on the opposite side, the antagonist, will usually lengthen and weaken. The inhibited (weak) muscle isn't then strong enough to carry out its normal functions, and other synergistic muscles will have to overwork to compensate. This is known as synergistic dominance. Synergistically dominant muscles are most susceptible to strains.

Stabilization of joints becomes more difficult due to a lengthening and weakening of the muscles and the lengthening of the ligamentous structures. Further compensations occur in the body to maintain balance over the base of support, and this can

again lead to any of the above factors. So let us take a look at each postural type in detail and highlight the potential problems it can cause.

Kyphosis

With a kyhosis posture, the steep angle of the sternum will restrict the diaphragm, reducing the amount of oxygen able to enter the lungs. This will limit athletes in their sport and manual workers in their work. Faulty breathing can also alter the body's delicate pH balance. When the pH of the blood is out of its normal range, a process begins that can potentially lead to many different diseases.

A kyphotic posture will also limit the amount of flexion available at the shoulder joint, as the head of the humerus hits against the acromium process of the scapula before the arm is fully flexed. In between the head of the humerus and the acromium process are the tendons of the biceps brachii and the supraspinatus muscles. With overhead movements such as those used in racket sports, swimming, and any job in which you carry materials overhead, these tendons are susceptible to entrapment and, therefore, sprains.

As mentioned previously, with a kyposis posture, the head migrates forward. When this happens, it increases the tension on the muscles of the neck. The farther forward the head migrates, the more work the neck muscles have to do to keep the head up. This creates a lot of tension in the muscles of the neck and upper back, which wastes a lot of energy and can make someone feel exhausted during the day. It can also

restrict blood flow to the brain and cause headaches.

Lordosis

With a lordosis posture, the zygopophyseal joints of the spine are closer together than is ideal. Therefore, with movements that create spinal extension or rotation, these joints approximate much earlier than normal and place more stress on each other than is normal. Over time, if this excessive stress continues, one or more of these joints can fracture. This type of fracture is called a spondylolysis. This fracture can become worse and can eventually completely break. This then causes the vertebra to "slip" forward and a clear ridge can be felt in the spine where the slippage occurs. This type of break is called a spondylolysthesis. A spondylolysthesis can also cause what is called a stenosis (blockage). With a stenosis, the spinal canal, which houses the spinal cord, becomes restricted. The spinal cord can then be irritated by the bone, causing the stenosis and leading to pain locally and down into the arms or legs.

With these types of injuries, pain is normally increased with spinal extension. If you suspect either a spondylolysis or a spondylolysthesis, you should seek professional advice.

A lordosis posture normally coincides with an anterior pelvic tilt. The anterior pelvic tilt can create:

- An internal rotation of the femur
- Lengthening of the abdominal muscles
- Lengthening of the gluteus maximus, medius, and hamstrings
- Sciatica

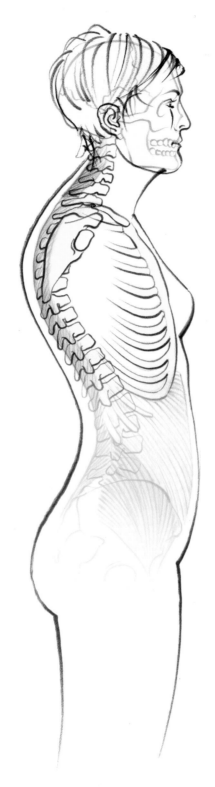

Kyphosis

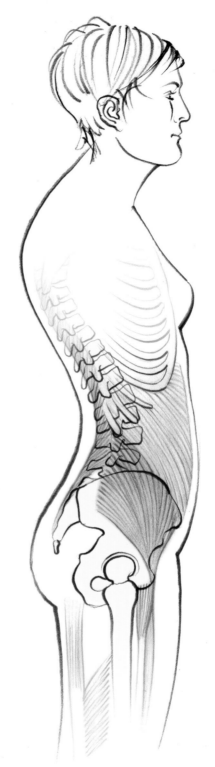

Lordosis

With an anterior rotation of the pelvis, the knees adduct and place stress on the medial side of the knee during movement, unless the abdominals and hip extensor muscles (gluteals and hamstrings) are strong enough to counteract this internal rotation. Because the abdominals and hip extensors are lengthened and therefore weakened, they are often unable to stabilize the knee. The knee is then more vulnerable to medial collateral and cruciate ligament sprain and cartilage tears.

As the knee adducts, it also translates weight onto the medial part of the foot and ankle, creating pronation of the ankle and eversion of the foot. This can lead to ankle sprains, achilles tendonitis, shin splints, and plantar fasciitis.

With a lengthening of the abdominal muscles, the normal stabilizing role of the abdominals is reduced. The abdominals help to stabilize the pelvis and the rib cage. This is particularly important as the pelvis is the foundation for the legs, and the rib cage is the foundation for the arms via the shoulder girdle (scapula and clavicle). Without proper stabilization of the limbs, the probability of any type of injury in the limbs is greatly increased.

The lengthening of the gluteals is important not just because it increases the probability of injuries in the legs, as stated above. With lengthened and weakened gluteals due to an anterior pelvic tilt, the hamstrings have to work harder during movement. One of the roles of the gluteus maximus is to help stabilize the sacroiliac joint (the joint between the sacrum and the ilium of the pelvis). This is essential during gait (walking, jogging, running, and sprinting), as all the weight of the upper body has to be stabilized through the sacroiliac, or SI, joint. The gluteus maximus during gait is the most powerful hip extensor that propels the body forward. The gluteus maximus also works in tandem with the latissimus dorsi on the opposite side to put tension through the thoracolumbar fascia to help stabilize the SI joint. If the gluteus maximus is weak, the biceps femoris (and other hip extensors) will have to work harder to extend the hip and will have to contract harder to stabilize the SI joint via the sacrotuberous ligament. This overworking of the hamstrings, in particular the biceps femoris, often leads to hamstring strains in athletes.

With the pelvis in anterior rotation, the piriformis muscle becomes stretched and taut. This brings the piriformis muscle and the sciatic nerve together, which can cause sciatica, a radiating pain down the posterior aspect of the legs.

Any spinal posture that is less than optimal will also restrict optimal rotation in the spine. The zygopophyseal joints will approximate sooner, which can cause problems and lead to sprains and strains in the spinal tissues.

Flat back

With a flat-back posture, the intervertebral disks are pressurized anteriorly. This anterior pressure pushes the disk posteriorly toward the spinal cord. The disk can "bulge" (commonly called a slipped disk), protruding beyond the vertebral body and entrapping the spinal nerve roots. This entrapment may or may not cause pain. This type of pain radiates into the legs and is called radicular pain.

As a flat-back posture normally comes with posterior rotation of the pelvis, the piriformis muscles tighten and can irritate the sciatic nerve and cause sciatic pain.

Any spinal posture that is less than optimal will also restrict optimal rotation in the spine. This can also lead to sprains and strains in the spinal tissues.

Sway back

A sway-back posture is a combination of the postures above, particularly the kyphosis and flat-back postures. It is therefore safe to suggest that a sway-back posture has the potential to lead to the same problems as caused by those postural problems.

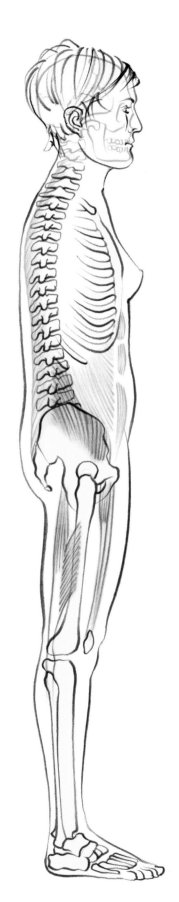

Flat back

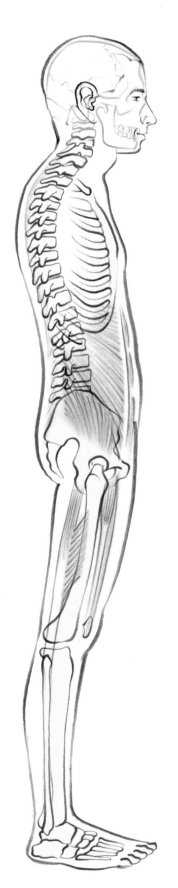

Sway back

When looking at the link between yoga and posture, we should consider posture in the context of symmetry: if we can balance the muscle groups, there is a likelihood that the posture will self-correct. If muscular balance is attained, excessive strain and stress on the system will dissipate and there will be an increase in proprioception (stimuli that are produced and perceived within an organism, especially those connected with the position and movement of the body) and energy efficiency as well as an improved sense of well-being. We will focus here on three of the main ways that yoga can help improve posture.

Increasing strength

When practicing the poses in yoga, we become aware of the imbalances in strength and flexibility unilaterally. Posture is about creating balance within the musculature. By increasing strength within the postural muscles (also known as tonic or type-I muscle), symmetry can be achieved. Due to the nature of yoga, each posture is held for one to three minutes. Research shows that the most effective way to strengthen tonic muscles is to hold a muscular contraction for up to three minutes. A common misconception of yoga is that it is all about increasing flexibility and nothing more. Each posture approached actually requires a combination of flexibility, strength, and endurance in order to hold the pose.

Improving flexibility

Yoga does far more than just increase our flexibility; it releases tensions and patterns from our mind and bodies. When approaching flexibility from a typical Western standpoint, flexibility reflects the ability to move muscles and joints through their complete range of motion, with no mention of flexibility in the mind. There are two schools of thought on how to increase physical flexibility, both of which can be applied to yoga and the practice of asana, a posture adopted in hatha yoga.

The first is to work to increase the flexibility of the connective tissue. This can be done by holding a stretch for a period of between 90 seconds and three minutes or longer. Holding a stretch for this period of time will allow the neuro-muscular system time to reprogram itself. If you were to hold the stretch for a shorter period of time, you would get a nice sense of release, but this would not allow for any profound structural changes—the muscular system would just return to its original length. When holding the posture for a long period of time, we are also working to enlist neurological mechanisms to assist with the release of tension. This is known as "reciprocal inhibition." Whenever there is one set of muscles working (agonist), there is a neurological process that causes the opposing muscle groups (antagonists) to release. This mechanism has always been used within yoga. For instance, in uttanasana (a standing forward bend), we contract the thigh muscles as we fold forward to release the hamstrings.

The second way to increase physical flexibility is through a technique known as "muscle energy technique" or MET. This uses a technique of muscle contraction and relaxation. For instance, if you are in the supine foot toe pose (see pages 104–105) and using a strap to hold the leg straight, by holding the strap taut and pressing your leg to the floor but not allowing the leg to move, you will contract the hamstrings. The intention is to hold this for up to eight seconds, then completely relax the hamstring and draw the leg back into the stretch. This can then be repeated a further two or three times. Although this is not a traditional practice within yoga, it can be used to help make improvements in particular postures. It is said that postural muscles respond well to this type of stretching.

Increasing body awareness

When we first come to yoga, our minds are occupied with achieving the correct alignment within the posture. Throughout the entire practice we are reminded to breathe well and maintain length in the spine. We start to cultivate an increased awareness of the physical feelings and differences from one side to the other. This new information that arises within us starts to awaken our minds as to how our bodies are in space; we start to become more conscious of our posture and find ourselves shifting our bodies to create the ideal alignment, not just on our yoga mats but in our daily lives.

The further we progress into our practice, the more our ability to listen to our body's internal messages develops. You may find, as you are standing or sitting in a pose for a long time, a feeling of frustration, anger, or joy may surface. More often than not we blame this feeling on the pose—"I really dislike this pose," or "I'm no good at this pose." When these thoughts arise, we are asked to look deeper, past the thought to the blockage to which it may be related. In yoga we practice how to hone our skills, in watching and witnessing these shifts within the body and then, importantly, letting them go.

THE BIOMECHANICS OF BREATH

The charts below introduce the muscular function of breath. Although there is an action described for each muscle, it is difficult to express what capacity of involvement they have—due to the level of activity the individual might be undertaking at any one time, breathing can be significantly altered not only by the level of activity but by the emotional state, postural position, health, and even the garments he or she may be wearing. Another issue to take into account when reading the charts is that the muscles listed may not act only in a singular capacity; for instance, the abdominals assist both inhalation and exhalation, and the diaphragm is also active in exhalation, although not in a huge capacity. The information gathered helps provide a clearer view of the muscular action during each cycle of the breath: this way we come to understand how posture and breath are interrelated. If we want to improve posture, we must also look at our breathing pattern, as this can have a detrimental effect on our posture, creating tension through the accessory muscles.

Muscles of inhalation

Primary muscles	Action
Diaphragm	Separates the thoracic and abdominal cavities. During inhalation, the muscle contracts and the dome descends into the abdominal cavity, decreasing the pressure of the thoracic cavity and allowing the lungs to fully expand. During exhalation, the diaphragm relaxes, increasing the pressure in the thoracic cavity
Levator costarum	Elevates and abducts the ribs, as well as laterally flexing the vertebral column
External intercostals	Stabilizes and maintains the shape and integrity of the rib cage. They elevate the ribs and expand the chest
Internal intercostals, anterior	Stabilizes and maintains the shape and integrity of the rib cage. They elevate the ribs and expand the chest

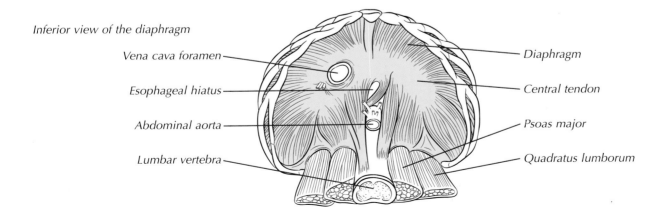

Inferior view of the diaphragm

Vena cava foramen

Esophageal hiatus

Abdominal aorta

Lumbar vertebra

Diaphragm

Central tendon

Psoas major

Quadratus lumborum

Muscles of inhalation (continued)

Accessory muscles	Action
Scalene	The anterior, medial and posterior scalenes elevate and firmly fix the first and second ribs during deep inhalation. They have also been observed being active during calm breathing
Sternocleidomastoid	Elevates the sternum, increasing the diameter of the chest
Trapezius	The upper trapezius helps elevate the thoracic cage during forced inspiration
Serratus anterior and serratus posterior superior	The serratus anterior is active in forced inspiration when the scapula is in adduction, fixing the insertion; it helps expand the rib cage by pulling the insertion to the origin. The serratus posterior superior expands the chest
Latissimus dorsi	The posterior fibers of the latissimus dorsi that are active during trunk extension are also believed to assist with inhalation
Subclavicus	The action of the subclavicus is to draw the clavicle down and stabilize it. This suggests that the muscle is important in the avoidance of clavicular breathing
Pectoralis major and minor	The pectoralis major is active when the arms and shoulders are fixed; the muscle can then use its insertion as an origin and lift the ribs and sternum. The pectoralis minor assists in forced inspiration, lifting the ribs if the scapula is fixed
Erector spinae, thoracic	Aids in inhalation by extending the thoracic spine, raising the rib cage

(adapted from F. Kendall et al, *Muscles: Testing and Function*)

Muscles of exhalation

Primary muscles	Action
Internal obliques	Especially active toward the end of the exhalation. The lower fibers contract significantly to raise the intra-abdominal pressure to meet the demands of, and increase, breath pattern
External obliques	Assist to reduce fluctuations within the thoracic cage volume and help maintain constancy of pressure
Rectus abdominus	Acts in conjunction with the obliques and transverses in exhalation
Tranversus abdominus	Especially active toward the end of the exhalation. The lower fibers contract significantly to raise the intra-abdominal pressure to meet the demands of, and increase, breath pattern
Internal intercostals, posterior	The posterior portion of the internal intercostals depress the ribs and act during exhalation
Transversus thoracis	Also acts to decrease the volume in the thoracic cavity and also narrows the chest by depressing the ribs from the second to the sixth

(adapted from F. Kendall et al, *Muscles: Testing and Function*)

Accessory muscles	Action
Latissimus dorsi	The anterior fibers that are active in torso flexion are also active during exhalation
Serratus posterior inferior	Acts to draw the ribs back and downward
Qaudratus lumborum	During exhalation, fixes the posterior fibers of the diaphragm via the 12th rib, preventing it from being elevated
Iliocastlis lumborum	Not a strong accessory muscle, but as it is attached to the sixth or seventh lower ribs, it has a possibility of assisting

(adapted from F. Kendall et al, *Muscles: Testing and Function*)

Changes in rib cage dimensions during breath

Rib cage movement during breath

Inhalation

Inhalation

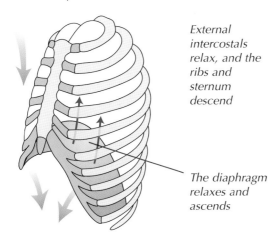

External intercostals contract to elevate the ribs and sternum

The diaphragm contracts and descends

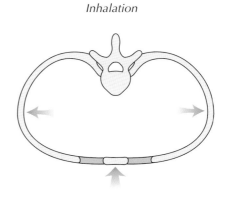

Expiration

Expiration

External intercostals relax, and the ribs and sternum descend

The diaphragm relaxes and ascends

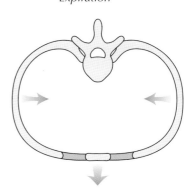

An interesting fact that is often overlooked is the size of the lungs and the large capacity that they have to exchange gases. The most superior part of the lungs starts just underneath the clavicle and finishes with the most inferior part, which sits on the diaphragm. It is said that we only use about one third of the capacity of our lungs, and this can be due to paradoxical breathing patterns.

The diaphragm is very much like a piston. As you inhale, the dome-shaped muscle contracts and descends downward toward the abdominal cavity. This expands the circumference of the rib cage and decreases pressure within the thoracic cavity, drawing air into the lungs and allowing them to expand to their full capacity. As the diaphragm descends, it increases the pressure in the abdominal cavity, pushing the organs down and forward slightly from their anatomical resting position; this action massages the abdominal organs, helping them maintain their motility.

During exhalation, the diaphragm relaxes and recoils into the thoracic cavity, mildly compressing the heart and lungs and reducing the expansion of the rib cage. As this movement occurs, the pressure in the abdominal region reduces, drawing the abdominal contents back and in toward the spine.

Breathing diaphragmatically supplies the maximum amount of air possible to the lungs with the minimum amount of effort. It also has a direct effect on the internal organs, especially the digestive system.

Breathing patterns

Respiration is often divided into four groups. Diaphragmatic breathing is the breath pattern that is used most during a hatha yoga practice. The rhythmical movements of this breathing pattern directly affect the central nervous system, creating a sense of calm and ease. It can also help maintain a meditative state throughout the practice. An individual who breathes diaphragmatically will be calm and balanced in demeanor and will handle stressful situations well.

Abdominal breathing

This particular breathing pattern is best used during relaxation periods. During inhalation, the rib cage stays relatively still and just the abdominal area lifts and falls. Unlike the diaphragmatic breath, which keeps the mind alert but calm, abdominal breathing calms the mind and draws you toward introspection, making it an effective breathing pattern during relaxation poses, such as the corpse pose.

Diaphragmatic inhalation

During diaphragmatic inhalation (see illustration, right) the diaphragm presses down onto the abdominal organs and the lower abdominal wall stays relatively still. This can be due to muscular resistance, standing, sitting, or both in combination, when the bottom of the rib cage is flared. This breathing can create a mental state of clarity and alertness.

Reverse breathing pattern

Faulty posture and increased stress and anxiety within our lives are affecting the patterns of our respiration. We spend longer hours at work sitting at a desk hunched over a computer, our minds constantly busy with thoughts of activities we have to complete; there is little room for connecting with our breathing patterns. As a result, reverse breathing patterns have become prevalent. This is when the diaphragm stays relaxed during inhalation and exhalation (see diagram opposite). The external intercostals and the accessory muscles of inhalation lift the rib cage, diaphragm, and the abdominal contents, sucking in the abdomen. During exhalation, the abdomen moves back out as the rib cage and abdominal contents return.

The problem with this type of breathing pattern is that it stimulates the sympathetic nervous system, which is the body's natural "fight or flight" response. It can create a stress response within the body, which will have a direct effect on the endocrine system. The endocrine system is responsible for the hormones that are released within the body.

Another result of this type of breathing is that the accessory muscles of inhalation are more active than is necessary, creating excessive tension in the neck and shoulder region, which is a common complaint.

Any individuals with a reversed breathing pattern may also suffer from symptoms of anxiety and stress.

Reversed inhalation

In reversed inhalation (see illustration, far right) the diaphragm is lifted but relaxed, the upper chest is at maximal expansion lifted by the external intercostals, and the abdominal wall is sucked in passively. This can cause the mental state to become anxious and agitated.

Thoracic breathing

Thoracic breathing is another common breathing pattern, which tends to be a precursor to the reverse breathing pattern. During a thoracic breath, the diaphragm remains still as you inhale and the abdominal wall is held taut by muscular action. The external intercostal muscles actively lift the chest up and out, and the rib cage will expand but not to its full capacity due to the tension in the abdominal wall. During exhalation, the chest will drop but the abdomen will continue to stay relatively taut.

Unfortunately, we are in a society where physical appearance holds great importance. This can sometimes have a positive effect, but when

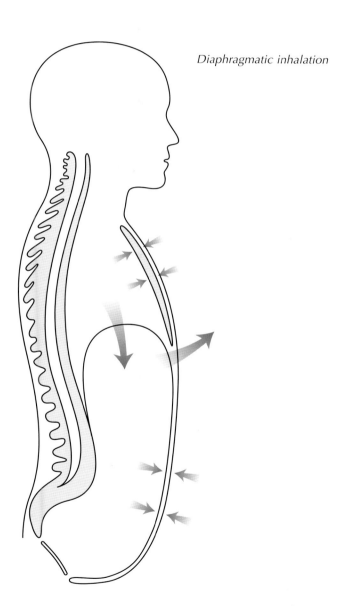

Diaphragmatic inhalation

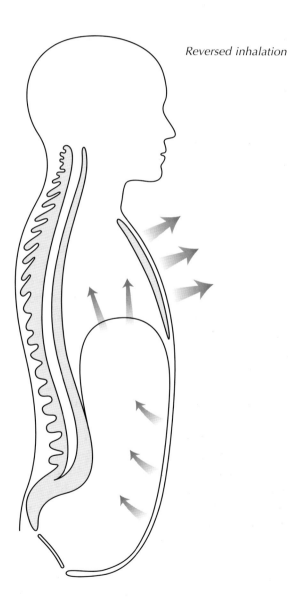

Reversed inhalation

it comes to the abdominal area, it can have a negative impact. Individuals find it incredibly difficult to relax the stomach area, finding themselves constantly pulling in their stomachs to create the illusion of a flatter stomach. Continuous repetitions of this action can create a faulty breathing pattern. This is not to say that it is wrong to draw in the stomach, especially when embarking on a physical activity that requires strength from your core, but to constantly engage the abdominal musculature will force the breath to move higher into the rib cage.

Habitual chest breathing, as it is also known, will over time create mental and physical problems. It will chronically overstimulate the sympathetic nervous system, possibly creating blood pressure issues and difficulties in digestion and elimination.

THE SYNERGY OF YOGA AND BREATH

Yoga without the connection of breath awareness is simply a stretching practice, something not too dissimilar from gymnastics. What separates yoga from other physical forms of exercise or body movement is breath mindfulness. An important aspect of yoga is the strengthening and cultivating of one's life force, also known in Sanskrit as *prana*. The ancient yogis, who spent years in the Himalayan mountains, observed that the life span of living creatures was determined according to their respiration rate. Cats and dogs breathe around 40 breaths per minute, and their life span is 10 to 20 years. Other animals such as elephants and tortoises have a far longer life span. For instance, the giant tortoise has a respiration rate of four breaths per minute, and they can live to 300. Yogis realized that the ability to have control over our breathing patterns will have a direct effect on our longevity and vitality. They also knew that a disturbed breathing pattern can have a direct effect on the fluctuations within our minds. As Muktibodhananda said in *Hatha Yoga Pradipika*, "When

prana (breath) moves, chitta (the mental force) moves. When prana is without movement, chitta is without movement. By this (steadiness of prana) the yogi attains steadiness."

The breathing process is directly connected to the central nervous system. It is the most vital process we have: without breath, there is no life. We can survive without food and water for a short time, but not breath. Breathing patterns also have a connection to the hypothalamus, the main brain control center for the autonomic nervous system, coordinating heart activity, blood pressure, body temperature, water balance, and endocrine activity. It also contains the centers that deal with emotional states and biological actions. The hypothalamus is active in transforming the mental process of perception.

Interestingly, within the hypothalamus there is an area known as "the pleasure center": "The pleasure center reinforces our drives to eat, drink, and procreate, but in doing so it also makes us perilously vulnerable. Few would deny that much of what we do and value is driven by the 'pleasure prin-

ciple'." (E. Marieb, *Human Anatomy and Physiology*)

Improving our breathing patterns has a direct effect on our physical and emotional states. The aim of the practices within this book are to encourage a personal connection with your breath and an understanding of its movements and capabilities, along with the effects that occur as you change your breathing patterns. Within the yogic texts there are many breathing practices also known as "pranayama" (life force; "yama" means control). For more information on different practices, please refer to the further reading on page 139.

Breath and movement
During an asana (pose) practice there are certain rules that apply as to when one should inhale and exhale—each movement that is completed should align with the breath, whether it is an inhalation or an exhalation (see tables, opposite). The intention when merging a movement with the breath is to allow each movement to last the entirety of the breath. So, for example, as you start an inhalation, start to lift your arms upward. As you finish the

Inhalation movements

Action of inhalation	Description of movement
Extension of spine and limbs	When lifting arms upward Straightening legs/arms Lifting up from a prone position on the floor Coming to standing
Moving to the center	Moving back to the center from a seated twist Moving back to center from a side bend

Exhalation movements

Action of exhalation	Description of movement
Flexion of spine and major limbs	When returning arms from extension Bending legs/arms Lowering yourself to the floor Lying down Coming up from lying to sitting Bending forward
Moving to the center	Moving away from the center in a seated twist Moving away from the center during a side bend

inhalation, the movement should finish, and as you start your exhalation, the arms start their journey back, and finish when the exhalation is completed.

Breath awareness should be constant, and, when holding a pose, the mind should be directed to the quality of the breath. If, for instance, you are in a standing pose that you find challenging, the breath may start to become erratic—this is an indicator that you are pushing yourself too hard. As we learned earlier, if the breath becomes erratic, the fluctuations of the mind will increase, and eventually the pose will become a struggle. By maintaining a smooth, even breath, we will be more likely to attain "sukha" (the ability to remain comfortable in a posture) and "sthira" (steadiness and alertness) within each pose for the entire practice. This is the goal of yoga: to find complete union of breath, mind, and body.

To help understand what meditation is, we will start by looking at the way in which modern psychology has categorized the different compartments of the mind. The unconscious and the subconscious can be divided into three groups: the lower mind, the middle mind, and the higher mind. The lower mind is concerned with bodily functions, such as circulation, respiration, and the functioning of the internal organs. It is also from this part of the mind that thoughts of self-doubt and self-worth arise, along with fear and phobias. These deep-seated issues feed the middle mind, which can manifest itself as emotions, such as anger and jealousy.

The middle mind is related to understanding incoming information during our waking state. It is this part of the mind that analyzes and reacts to outside influences, solves problems, and answers questions that arise within. This is the domain of cognitive thinking.

The higher mind is the area of supreme consciousness; this is the area of the mind that relates to moments of inspiration, intuition, flashes of genius, and creativity. It is the source of deeper knowledge.

We spend our time largely within the middle mind, conscious only of a small part of the mind's infinite capabilities and activities. But behind all of these different functioning planes is our true essence, the center of our being, our true self: it is this we hope to awaken during meditation, tapping into the different areas of the mind and opening the doors of intuitive knowledge. When we meditate, we are able to take our consciousness out of the realms of the middle mind, to move away from judging and intellectualization and into a state of inner peace and tranquillity.

To start the journey of meditation, we must first learn to focus the mind on one point. This at first seems easy, but once sitting and settling ourselves, we soon understand that the mind has a lot to think about: issues of the day ahead and thoughts concerning past actions that tend to have no relevance to the present moment. So the first stage of meditation is to master the art of one-pointed focus, to harness the mind to stay present. This can be done with your breath, a picture, a sound, or a mantra. A mantra is a syllable or poem, typically in Sanskrit, that is used to instill focus. The mantra can either be done with verbal repetition, creating a vibration throughout the body, or it can be an internal mental incantation. Focusing on these subjects helps divert the mind away from basic instinctual desires or material inclinations.

Once success has been mastered in this stage and you are able to maintain a calm and introverted mind, there will be a natural progression to the free flow of thoughts, visions, and memories from the deepest realms of the unconscious lower mind. At this point one works to become a witness, watching these thoughts arise as if watching a movie screen, acknowledging lovingly and with acceptance the emotions that may arise with the thought, but not allowing yourself to get caught up in the "movie." This is the time in which we learn more about our patterns in life: why we act in a certain way when someone confronts us; how we communicate with loved ones; and what it is exactly that gets us so annoyed. The challenge at this point is to be able to acknowledge all these revelations and then manage to let them go. Now that they have been brought into your consciousness, it is time to rid yourself of them, resisting the urge to become a victim of them.

Once the lower mind has been explored and cleansed, you move into the supreme consciousness of the higher mind. Here we can tap into the infinite knowledge that is stored within us, awaken to our natural intuitive capabilities, and enjoy a constant stream of creativity: here, deep mediation begins. Beyond this point we transcend the mind, becoming one with supreme consciousness and self-realization.

As Buddha said, "Meditation brings wisdom; lack of meditation leaves ignorance. Know well what leads you forward and what holds you back and choose the path that leads to wisdom." Meditation is a wonderful journey of self-discovery, but one must not crave the end goal or desire self-realization: to get caught in this circle of thought will move you further away. One must sit and practice for the pure joy of it—the joy of self–discovery: "Meditation is experiencing oneself in stillness." (E. Schiffmann, *Yoga: The Spirit and Practice of Moving Into Stillness*).

The meditation practices that have been chosen for this book are aimed at the first stages of meditation, teaching the mind to become focused. It is best to seek out an experienced teacher if you wish to further your understanding and practice of meditation.

Benefits

There are many styles of meditation practice and plenty of scientific research has been carried out on its effects, and the overall evidence is overwhelming. Meditation will improve your health and well-being. The profound effects of meditation on your mind and internal dialogue can be improved significantly, which will, in turn, improve self-esteem, confidence, and self-worth. The benefits of regular meditation are endless, so the following are just a few that have been found through scientific research:

- Decreased insomnia
- Increased personal development
- Decreased stress and anxiety
- Reduced risk of cardiovascular-related deaths
- Lowered blood pressure
- Improved ability to focus and concentrate
- Improved moods
- Improved memory
- Increased sense of calm and control
- Helps to create a state of deep relaxation
- General feeling of well-being

Meditation posture

For many people in the Western industrialized world, sitting involves some form of chair, often a comfortable sofa. Very rarely would the thought of sitting with crossed legs to eat our evening meal or to read a book occur to us, and because of this fact most of us suffer from a lack of flexibility in the pelvis, legs, and back, physically preventing us from sitting on the floor. With this in mind, it is important to find a sitting posture that is comfortable. If you find that after a few minutes of sitting certain areas of your body start to complain, this will draw your focus away from your meditation. You may find that you can ignore this discomfort for a while and force yourself to sit through the pain, but sooner or later it will nag at you until you have to stop meditating. As previously mentioned, you should sit and meditate for the joy of sitting and meditating, and if this means practicing while sitting on a chair to start with, then that should be your posture.

The body's role in mediation is to support the mind, freeing it up to focus on one point. Ideally, it will be in a position that you are able to maintain comfortably, that does not create tension in the lower or upper back, and that allows a deep sense of relaxation. For the practices chosen in this book, the aim is to sit in stillness. Since the mind needs to be alert, it is ideal to keep the body upright: if one lies down, the tendency to become drowsy and nod off is highly likely. The body should be in a position that uses the least amount of energy to maintain—this way the heart can be at its quietest and the breath can be both unrestricted and smooth.

Ideal postural alignment

Whether sitting on the floor with or without support, or on a chair, ideal postural alignment is an integral part of the meditation practice. The pelvis has to be in a neutral position, slumping neither too far forward into an anterior tilt nor too far backward into a posterior tilt. With the pelvis in neutral, the spine should be erect, maintaining all of its natural curves. The neck and head should be in line with the center of the pelvic basin, and the shoulders should be relaxed and in line with the ears. Your body weight needs to be evenly distributed between the sitting bones, and therefore balanced and symmetrical throughout the spine.

Pain

One obvious indication of poor alignment in sitting is pain. Certainly some aches and pains are best ignored, as are itches or the general need to fidget—some of the time these are more likely linked to an unsettled mind, therefore creating a diversion from stillness. By allowing yourself to become involved with this restlessness, you will not connect with your meditation, and it is important to acknowledge that this may be the root of your discomfort. But it is also important to be sensitive when assessing your discomfort: you should not be experiencing numbness or pins and needles in your limbs. If sharp pain arises, this is another indicator to come out of the posture; pain that increases the more you sit is also a warning sign. Our bodies are precious, and we must honor them by practicing meditation with alertness and compassion.

Sukhasana (easy crossed-leg sitting)

Sukhasana is one of the most comfortable sitting positions when starting, but if you suffer from tightness, it may feel difficult to sit with an erect spine for any length of time. Placing a block underneath your buttocks, as in the illustration overleaf, can help keep the pelvis in a neutral position. The best way to make sitting on a block or blanket effective is to slide your sitting bones off the edge of the support and leave the muscle on it.

Kneeling

If sitting is proving painful or uncomfortable, kneeling may be easier. To help keep your back straight, you may need to sit on a cushion or on your haunches, so that your hips are slightly raised above your knees.

Siddhasana

The sitting pose of siddhasana is said to direct energy from the lower chakras upward through the spine, stimulating the brain and calming the nervous system. This is due to the lower foot pressing toward the perenium—the area of the root chakra (mooladhara).

There are many other suitable seated poses, but for the purposes of this book, we have chosen to stay with the three shown.

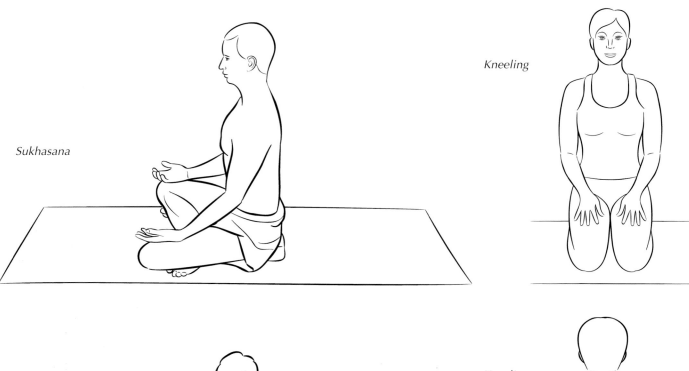

Sukhasana

Kneeling

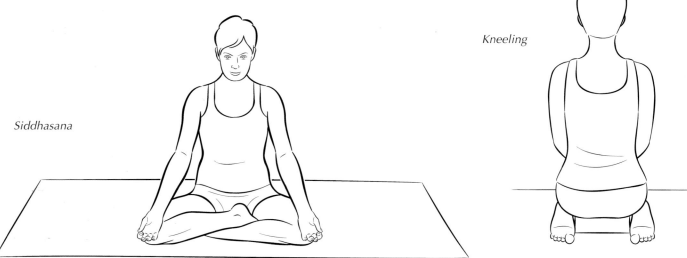

Siddhasana

Kneeling

THE CHAKRAS

Chakras, or the body's energy centers, are a complex subject, and one that is difficult to explain in such a short introduction. The intention is for you to understand the relationship between the chakras and certain behavioral patterns and postural imbalances. When embarking on the journey of self-discovery, or the journey of improving one's posture, all avenues to the end goal must be explored. This means not only practicing specific postural exercises, but also exploring spiritual, emotional, and mental issues. When we look at our physical body, we only look at how we can physically change it; what exercises can help us improve that particular problem. Very rarely do we think or even contemplate that our shoulders being rounded or our chest being collapsed may have some correlation to our low self-esteem or lack of self-confidence. By understanding the unwanted behavioral traits and emotional patterns that are related to specific chakras, we can start to contemplate, accept, and then let go of these patterns and move a step further along our evolutionary path.

Chakras are related to our body's subtle levels—life force (prana), knowledge (manas), understanding (buddhi), ego (ahamkara), and feeling (chitta). They are vortices through which energy flows in and out. There are thought to be seven major chakras, and they bridge the gap between the body's subtle level and the gross material level (flesh, bone, fat, marrow, fluids, etc.). They are situated in a line from the perineum (the area between the genitals and anus) to the crown of the head,

embedded along a channel of energy known as a nadi. There are said to be 72,000 nadis within the body, channeling energy throughout. The concept of nadis is similar to that of meridian lines in Chinese medicine and acupuncture.

The word "chakra" comes from the Sanskrit word meaning "wheel" or "disk," and from this we can visualize them spinning and vibrating as the prana moves through them. They are often depicted as lotus flowers, which are seen as the flowers of transformation—their journey to full bloom goes through mud and water and then finally into the air, basking in the energy of the universe. This is very similar to the journey of humankind: as we evolve, we become more connected to the universe, but first we must travel through the material world and find our place within it.

Prana is the key to the functioning of the chakras. We are energetic beings surrounded by a bioelectromagnetic field, and from this field the chakras draw energy in or disperse it. If prana is flowing freely through the nadis and chakras, then the chakras will spin in harmony, creating a life of balance, calmness, and tranquillity, free from the burdens of past life issues. More often than not there will be energy blocks throughout our system; these can be anything from physical problems to emotional issues to environmental toxicity, or even poor diet. These blocks can affect the flow of energy. If one chakra has a blockage and its vibrational frequency slows down, this will precipitate the other chakras. The result can be a feeling of being stuck or restricted, a lack of drive and

enthusiasm, and even depression, so it is imperative that we work to bring harmony and balance back within our body, increasing our well-being and vitality.

Each chakra relates to a certain stage in our life, and during that stage we learn different lessons. If at any stage something happened to us, maybe physically or emotionally—a childhood drama, an emotional hurt, a physical injury—there is likely to be a lasting effect within one of the chakras. To move forward from this point, we have to first understand where we may have blocked physical or emotional memories, identify them, then release ourselves from them. By having a deeper awareness of the characteristics of unbalanced/balanced chakras, we can work to free ourselves from these issues.

The first chakra relates to our physical survival in this world (ages 1–7), the second relates to our relationship with our personal sexuality and our relationship to the opposite sex (ages 8–14), the third chakra relates to our personal power and self will (ages 14–21), the fourth relates to our ability to love and receive love and feel compassion and forgiveness (ages 21–28), the fifth is our ability to communicate (ages 28–35), the sixth is our ability to awaken to our inherent nature of creativity, wisdom, and intuition (age 35 onward), and finally the seventh chakra is our ongoing relationship with the universe and all that is within it.

Balancing the chakras

Increasing the prana within the body will help dislodge any blockages, and

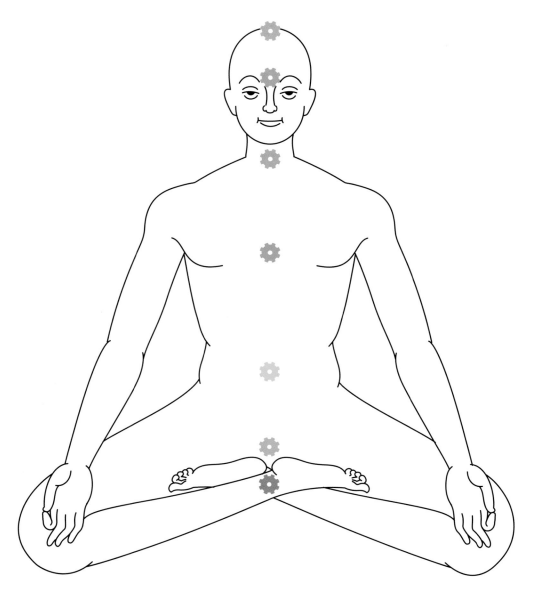

prana can be increased by improving your posture and breathing patterns. Improved posture allows the body to become more energy-efficient, and yoga postures (asanas) can achieve this. We can also use sound—each chakra has a *bija* mantra, a seed sound. This sound resonates with the natural frequency of each particular chakra, helping bring about balance. Visualization is also beneficial in generating prana to the chakras, by focusing on each chakra and visualizing its color radiating brightly. Focusing on a shape or pattern, known as a yantra, and reciting positive affirmations, are also powerful.

The following pages will describe the chakras in more detail. Some may resonate with you, whereas others may not. Approach each chakra with an open mind. At first you may not see a resemblance, but after thought and practice, you may unearth issues of which you were unaware.

Root chakra, muladhara

Chakra name	Location	Color	Element	Bija mantra	Associated body part
Root chakra: muladhara (mul = base, adhara = support)	Perineum, below the genitals, base of the spine, the pelvic plexus	Red	Earth	Lam	Bones, skeletal structure

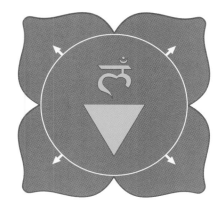

The first chakra is connected to the earth element and is related to our basic survival and safety needs. It relates to how we see ourselves in our surroundings. Do we have a secure and safe home life, are we happy in our home, in our financial status, in our relationships with family members? All these factors have a direct correlation to the root chakra. Infants tend to act out the root chakra. They are in a new world, a strange environment in which they need to test their boundaries. Their instincts for survival are prevalent, and they need to know that they are safe and secure within the family unit.

An unbalanced root chakra, which is low in vital energy, can manifest itself in the following characteristics: safety and security issues, a sense that the individual is unable to provide for life's necessities, ongoing dramas with family, low self-esteem, and emotional neediness. It can also lead to self-destructive behavior—smoking, alcoholism, drug addiction, or eating disorders. On a physical level, low back pain and sciatica can be experienced and possible immune system-related disorders and depression have also been connected.

When the root chakra is overactive, it can lead to bullying behavior, being overly materialistic, and having a self-centered approach to life.

When the chakra maintains equilibrium and spins at its correct vibrational speed, there will be a deep sense of security, both physically and mentally. Self-confidence will be high, physical energy and life force are attained, and there is fearlessness in meeting life's challenges.

Sacral chakra, svadhishthana

Chakra name	Location	Color	Element	Bija mantra	Associated body part
Sacral chakra: svadhishthana (sva = self or prana, adhishthana = dwelling place)	Lower abdomen, between the navel and genitals	Orange	Water	Vam	Sex organs, large intestine, lower vertebrae, pelvis, appendix, bladder, hip area

The second chakra is related to the element of water, and water is connected to life. By extension, this chakra is related to procreation, our fantasies, sexuality, and sensuality. The first chakra is about our relationships with family. The second chakra revolves around our relationships with friends and the opposite sex, where our intention is diverted to creativity and fantasies of a sexual nature.

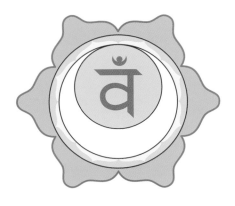

Children from the ages of 8–14 belong in this chakra—they are now established as people, which frees up time to explore friendships and physical contact. There are also changes to their physical body and a new awareness of their sexuality.

When the chakra's vibration is low, the individual can become over-sensitive, have feelings of guilt for no reason, feel unbalanced in life, and may start to seek satisfaction through outside influences, such as sex, food, and material possessions. Physical dysfunctions that may manifest are low back pain, sciatica and sexual potency issues, as well as possible urinary and gynecological problems.

If the chakra is too active, there is a lack of balance, issues related to a sexual nature can arise, and subjects may find themselves becoming manipulative.

When the chakra spins harmoniously the individual is trusting, expressive, has ethics and honor in relationships, and is creative in thought and action.

Solar plexus chakra, manipura

Chakra name	Location	Color	Element	Bija mantra	Associated body part
Solar plexus chakra: manipura (mani = jewel or gem, pura = dwelling place)	The part of the vertebral column that relates to the navel region, solar plexus	Yellow	Fire	Ram	Abdomen, stomach, upper intestines, liver, gallbladder, kidney, pancreas, adrenal glands, spleen, middle spine

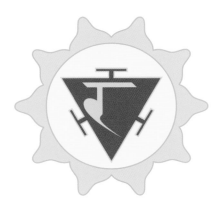

The third chakra is located at the navel center, the seat of our emotions. This chakra relates to how we perceive ourselves within society and involves taking ownership for the choices we make in the face of life's challenges. Young adults between the ages of 14–21 belong in the third chakra—this is the time of individual identification, of becoming confident in choices made and of separating themselves from family rules and constraints. This age group is concerned with what they wear as an expression of themselves, with current fashion trends playing a strong role. With the first chakra, we are governed by our family, the second chakra involves the discovery of the opposite sex, and with the third chakra we become controlled by our need for personal power.

Named the solar plexus chakra, its relationship is with the fire element, which can manifest itself in a determination to achieve—the phrase "a burning desire" is relevant to this chakra. This energy also governs the digestive system: if unbalanced colon and intestinal problems arise, chronic indigestion and dysfunction in the adrenals and liver can also appear.

If a low vibrational frequency occurs, the individual may become overly concerned with what people think, therefore living by another person's goals and ambitions. The individual will look for constant reassurance, hoping that the decisions made were the right ones. Is your self-perception right? Are you a nice person? A deep insecurity develops in personal abilities and choices.

If the chakra is too open, the opposite can occur. People can become overly driven to control their environment to the detriment of others, even their family and friends. They can become judgmental, overpowering and anger easily.

When balanced, the individual will reach a deep level of self-acceptance and self-respect. They will have the ability to take risks and make decisions, with the knowledge that any obstacle that presents itself can be handled. This is the true essence of personal power.

Heart chakra, anahata

Chakra name	Location	Color	Element	Bija mantra	Associated body part
Heart chakra: anahata (unstruck or unbeaten)	The heart region of the vertebral column, center of the chest	Green/pink	Air	Yam	Heart and circulatory system, lungs, shoulders and arms, ribs/ breasts, diaphragm, thymus gland

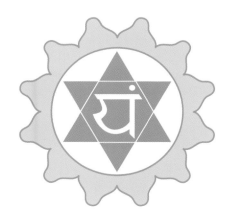

The heart chakra is concerned with balancing the love we have for others with the love we have for ourselves. It is at this stage that we discover that after all the exploration of the lower chakras, we may have neglected to understand and love every side of ourselves. We enter into relationships, giving us the perfect opportunity to learn about ourselves, the dark sides included. At this stage in life we learn to love unconditionally by building a solid foundation of self-intimacy and self-acceptance, an ability to forgive past hurts with compassion. From the ages of 21–28, we act from the heart space, coming to understand our life purpose, hopefully experiencing love and long-standing relationships.

When in balance, there is a deep love for ourselves that leads to the ability to love unconditionally. Being secure in one's own feelings means that one doesn't "need" to be loved. There is a radiance that surrounds the individual who is balanced in the heart; they are friendly, patient, and calm.

When overly active, individuals can find themselves professing "love" when really they are acting from an external place and not from within; there is jealousy, possessiveness, and emotional instability.

If the energy is low, individuals can become codependent, there is a "need" for love but when love comes there is an inability to receive it. There is often a fear of betrayal, one of the common emotional dysfunctions of the heart chakra, and fears of rejection can also arise.

Due to the location of the heart chakra, there is an association with the heart and lungs, so physical dysfunctions can arise within the circulatory system, lungs, and heart. There may also be heart issues, asthma, and breathing difficulties, along with issues related to the neck and shoulders.

Throat chakra, vishuddha

Chakra name	Location	Color	Element	Bija mantra	Associated body part
Throat chakra: vishuddha (shuddhi = to purify)	Centrally at the base of the neck, throat, carotid plexus	Blue	Ether	Ham	Throat, thyroid, trachea, neck vertebrae, mouth, teeth, and gums, esophagus, parathyroid, hypothalamus

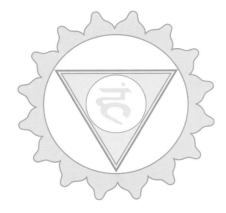

The throat chakra is the first of the chakras taking us toward our higher consciousness and into the realms of spirituality. Its connection is with our ability to communicate, be in touch with our inner voice, and be able to express verbally with compassion and acceptance our deepest feelings. We act from this chakra from the ages of 28 to 35.

When the throat chakra is in balance, you are able to enter into discussions with an open mind, but still maintain your own values and ideals. There is an ability to communicate hurt and anger in a way that does not disrespect the feelings of others. Individuals balanced in this chakra may find themselves in roles such as teachers or speakers, as they can communicate with enthusiasm and motivation.

When the chakra is sluggish in energy, the individual will be unable to express him or herself verbally and there will be an inability to communicate with others in a constructive and positive way. They may become tongue-tied or choose not to speak at all. This can create problems within the throat and neck area, such as laryngitis, neck pain, thyroid dysfunction, canker sores, and gum disease. They may speak with a raspy throat or in a dull, monotonous tone.

Conversely, if the chakra is overexcited, the individual may become overtalkative, generally speaking about nothing of interest. There may be an air of arrogance and self-righteousness.

Third eye chakra, ajna

Chakra name	Location	Color	Element	Bija mantra	Associated body part
Third eye chakra: ajna (the point at which the ajna chakra is based is called bhrumadhya—bru = eyebrow, madhya = center)	Above and between the eyebrows, medulla plexus, pineal plexus	Indigo	Light and telepathic energy	Om	Brain, nervous system, eyes, ears, nose, pineal gland, pituitary gland

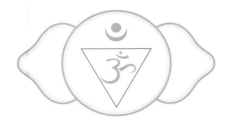

The sixth chakra is that of emotional intelligence; being able to open up to our inherent intuitive sight and wisdom. It involves the realization of non-duality, the union of mind, body, and spirit, and our connection with the universe and all that is in it. We are governed by the sixth chakra from the age of 35 onward.

The sixth chakra is where the solar and lunar energies meet. If balance occurs within this chakra, there are no mundane fluctuations of the mind and the challenges of the previous chakras have dissipated. Individuals have the confidence that all the answers to life's challenges lie deep within themselves. There is no fear when embarking on new ventures, just clarity, understanding, and excitement about the journey ahead. The need to meditate and contemplate is recognized in order to awaken their creative, intuitive side. At last there is no observed and no observer: they come to the realization that "I am that, that I am."

When out of balance, the individual will make choices out of fear, especially fear of failure. Individuals will not listen to their insights, or inner wisdom. They will listen to the negative chatter of the mind, which is frequently based on dramas and incidents that happened in the past and have no current relevance. These destructive thoughts tell them how ridiculous it is to even contemplate trying something creative and that they will only fail. Obstacles will be created to prevent them from succeeding, and they feel unworthy of success.

The location of the sixth chakra relates to areas around the brain and head, so if out of balance, problems with eyesight can occur as well as headaches and hearing problems. The possibility of learning difficulties can also arise.

Crown chakra, sahasrara

Chakra name	Location	Color	Element	Bija mantra	Associated body part
Crown chakra: sahasrara (dwelling place)	Top of the head, crown, cerebral plexus	White/gold/violet	Thought/cosmic energy	There is no seed sound; om can be used	Muscular system, skeletal system, skin

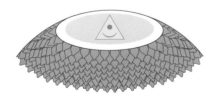

The seventh chakra is depicted as a thousand-petalled lotus flower at the crown of the head. This associates with the ultimate awakening and realization of the illusion of the "individual self." Sahasara is the seat of the self-luminous soul or the essence of being (H. Johari, *Chakras— Energy Center of Transformation*).

The seventh chakra is about opening ourselves up to the spirit of creation, living our lives through divine guidance, and seeing the world with a sense of wonder, love, amazement, and unity, as we did as a small child.

When you reach this ultimate balanced state, you are truly at peace with yourself and the world. You emanate love, wisdom, and compassion. Materialism and ego no longer rule. Some are even said to attain mystical powers (siddhis), but they have no desire to use them. They are magnetic.

When the chakra is blocked, there is a refusal to engage in or even believe in a higher consciousness. Life is filled with materialism, leaving you with thoughts such as, "Is this all my life is about?," not being able to see or find the true answer. You will be highly driven by your ego; you will realize that the sheer willpower that has carried you through life has no relevance to the true essence of life's purpose. This can lead to obsessional thinking, depression, and confusion, and sufferers may experience chronic exhaustion.

THE PRACTICE

The four sequences in this book have been created with the four specific postural types in mind, covering all the potential issues that may have contributed to any muscular imbalances.

There are five areas to cover within the entire sequence; it is ideal if you can complete each section in one practice, but it is not imperative. For instance, you could complete the breathing and meditation practice on their own at a different time—morning, for instance, would be the ideal time to set yourself up for the day. Each section of the sequence is effective in bringing about balance within the mind and body.

These days many people find it difficult to find spare time for themselves, so by spending a little time each day on the practice you will start to feel the benefits. If you can follow the full sequence three times per week, you are doing well. Alternatively, you could break up the practice into small segments; for instance, on day one: do contemplation, breathing practice, and meditation practice; then on day two: try contemplation, sun salutations, and the full sequence.

As you spend more time with the practice, you will awaken your intuition as to where the imbalances stem from. This will help you personalize the practice; you might feel that you want to spend more time on the meditation practice, for instance. It is important to seek a trained yoga teacher if you find that you want to clarify points in this book.

Related chakra focus

As we have already discovered, postural imbalances can cause energetic blockages in the chakras, and this section covers the possible chakras that may be blocked. After studying the chakras, you may have found other chakras that you feel you relate to. If so, keep those in mind. At the beginning of each practice come to a comfortable sitting position and spend a few moments contemplating the positive affirmations that are shown. Then try to cultivate a deep sense of gratitude and acceptance for these affirmations. You can also recite each bija mantra three to six times—this can be done verbally or mentally. Additionally, try to familiarize yourself with the locations and colors of the chakras, as this will help you direct energy through them. Spend at least five minutes at the beginning of the practice focusing on these points. This will help you become present and alert before starting the practice.

Sun salutations

The sun salutation has been introduced within this book as a warm-up prior to the asana (posture) practice; it is highly beneficial in warming the muscles and joints and is extremely energizing. If you have not practiced sun salutations before, three full rounds is a good starting point. As your strength and flexibility increase, move to between six and eight rounds. It is important to listen to your body when practicing—if you suffer from lower back pain, exercise

caution during the forward bends, be mindful of your knees, and if your wrists are stiff, use your fingers or knuckles.

The sequence

Each posture has been chosen to maximize the effect of attaining balance within the weak and tight areas of each specific postural imbalance. The sequence should be followed as shown in the book, as this will increase the effectiveness of each pose as well as the overall balance of the practice. In a traditional hatha yoga practice, each pose is completed once; due to the specific nature of this book, it would be more effective to complete each pose twice.

If you are a total beginner to yoga, complete each pose once until you build strength, then progress to holding the pose twice. Hold the first pose for between one minute and 90 seconds and hold the second pose from 90 seconds to two minutes. As you become stronger and more familiar with the poses, increase the length of holding time until you can hold for between two and three minutes for both poses. After each pose do the mountain pose (see page 48) for 10 to 20 breaths, then repeat. Try to allow your breathing to remain smooth and even and breath diaphragmatically.

Modifications have been included for progression into the postures; try the modifications first, and if you feel strong and open within the modification, then move on to the full pose.

Most importantly, you need to listen to your body. This is the way to prevent injury and strain to the muscles and joints. Be aware of the signals and messages that your body is sending you; resist the urge to override those signals. Approach each posture with the following stages in mind:

Stage one: when you start the pose, you may feel slight sensations as you align yourself.

Stage two: as you move further into the pose, you will experience your first muscle resistance barrier; it is here that you should hold.

Stage three: after holding for a few moments, slowly allow the body to release a little more; you may find that you move a little deeper into the asana. You should feel a stretch that takes your body into the outer edge of your comfort zone and then stop. If you experience pain, then you have taken your body into a danger zone.

Try to find a point of stillness within each pose and allow your mind to follow the wave of your breath, keep the body active and alert throughout each pose, and resist the inclination to become "floppy" or "sag" in the pose. Enjoy each pose for the joy of doing the pose, not for the outcome.

Breathing practice

There are four breathing practices in this book, each one relating to a particular postural imbalance. This is not meant to indicate that you shouldn't work with the other practices. On the contrary, it is encouraged that you try all the practices, as each one will have a positive effect in bringing union to the mind and body. Each practice will have a profound effect on improving your natural breathing patterns.

Meditation practice

Each meditation practice has been chosen to help balance the mental fluctuations of the mind. Meditation takes time and patience—sometimes you may sail through your meditation completely focused and present, but at other times your mind could be unruly and disruptive. The challenge is to accept whatever arises with compassion, laugh at the frustration that arises, smile at the stillness you achieve, and be joyful for the time you have to practice.

"Surya namaskar" means sun salutation. There are many variations of the sun salutation, but it is essentially a sequence of flowing movements that gently flex and extend the body in honor of the life-giving properties of the sun. It generates heat and openness within our physical form, allowing time to unite both the mind and body to the present moment. It creates space within us to transform and grow.

The flowing movements are most powerful when combined with the breath, which is shown here; the whole sequence then becomes a breath-led practice. If you have not practiced this sequence, it would definitely be beneficial to spend a few breaths within each asana, thereby familiarizing yourself with the correct alignment and the connection with your breath, which is a significant part of the practice. Daily practice will awaken, energize, and strengthen your entire being.

To further develop the sequence you have chosen, it is a good idea to prepare your body and mind before starting the sequence, and the sun salutation is the most profound way to do this. Complete it six to eight times before starting the practice. If you have more time, you can do more.

At all times you must practice safely, so sit before starting the practice and ask your inner teacher how many rounds your body would like to do—listen intently to the first answer that comes.

1. Mountain pose

- Keep your weight even between the balls and heels of your feet.
- Gently sense the lifting of the inner arches of your feet.
- Draw your inner thighs lightly together.
- Allow the coccyx to become heavy (do not do this if you are flat-back).
- Extend the crown of the head to the ceiling, drawing the chin back slightly.
- Draw the shoulder blades toward the spine and down, the middle finger of your hands in line with the seam of your shorts.
- Keep the front ribs from rising.

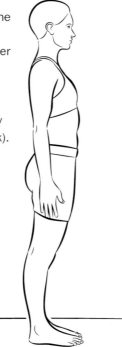

2. Mountain pose: raised arms (inhale)

- Maintain all the teaching points from the "mountain pose".
- Extend your arms to the ceiling, keeping the shoulder blades and front ribs engaged. Lift the upper chest slightly and look to the ceiling, maintaining length in the back of the neck.

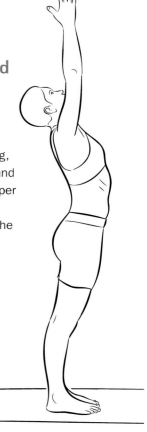

3. Forward bend (exhale)

- Keep your weight evenly on both feet and don't sway onto the balls or heels.
- Draw your navel in as you start to lower.
- Allow the upper inner thighs to move toward each other, bending your knees if necessary.
- Keep your shoulders moving away from your ears and keep the back of the neck lengthened.

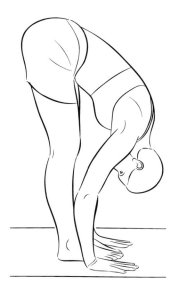

4. Lunge (inhale)

- Bend your knees deeply, place your hands on the floor, then lift the right leg and lunge it back as far as you can, then drop the knee to the ground.
- Your right knee should be directly over your right ankle—if it isn't, then adjust.
- With your arms on either side of your right leg, lift the upper chest and chin, maintaining the length in the back of the neck.
- Extend through the thoracic spine.

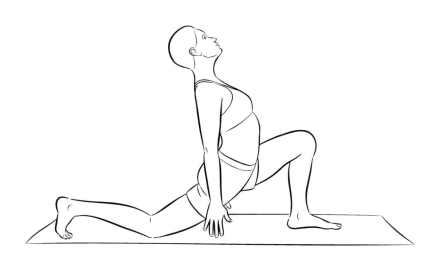

5. Plank (exhale)

- Ground your hands and step the left leg back to join the right. Bring the body into a straight line with your knees on the floor, pressing away with your heels.
- Draw your navel deeply into your spine to activate the transversus abdominis muscle.
- Your hands should be directly under your shoulders. Lower yourself to the ground with control, keeping the inner elbows and upper arms pressed into the side of the body, as if holding a piece of paper between them.
- If your legs are straight, then press your heels away from you. If this is too challenging and you feel you're losing form, drop your knees and deeply ground your hands and the balls of your feet.

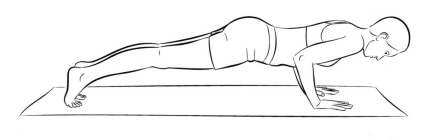

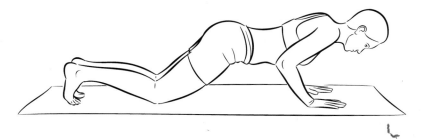

6. Cobra variation (inhale)

· Keep your hands underneath your shoulders.
· Press the tops of your feet to the floor, including the tops of the little toes.
· Press from your hands and lead with your chest, lifting your upper body but keeping your hips on the floor.
· As you lift, keep the shoulder blades anchored and the elbows drawn in to the outer edges of your rib cage.
· Try to maintain a smooth curve in your back and keep your gaze on the horizon or on the floor. In this variation of the cobra the back of the neck maintains length—try not to push the chin forward.

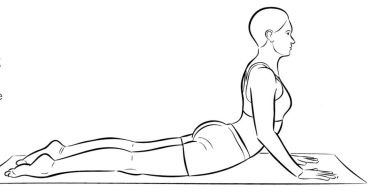

7. Down dog (exhale)

· Lower down from the cobra, then tuck the toes under, pressing back from your hands, especially the index finger and thumb base. Lift your sitting bones back and up to the ceiling, with your feet hip-width apart.
· Roll your biceps up to the ceiling, allowing your shoulders to move away from your ears, creating space and length for your neck. Allow your neck to completely relax and have the ears in line with the inner arms.
· Draw the sitting bones (ischial tuberosities) away from your heels and press the heels evenly to the floor. If your hamstrings are too tight, keep the heels off the floor and keep the focus on lifting the sitting bones.
· Stay in this position for five full breaths.

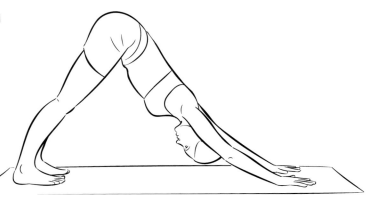

Return to

8. Lunge (inhale)

· Lift your head and look forward. As you inhale, step your right foot forward.

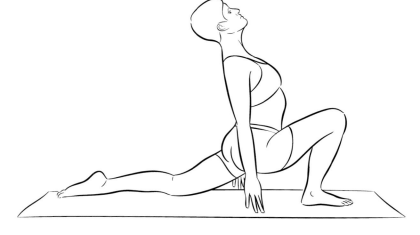

9. Forward bend (exhale)

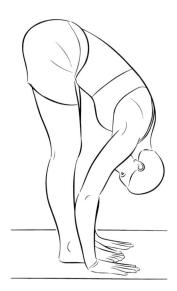

10. Mountain pose: raised arms (inhale)

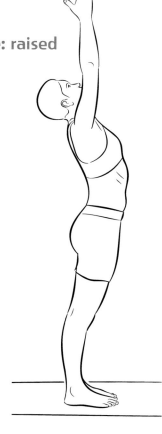

11. Mountain pose (exhale)

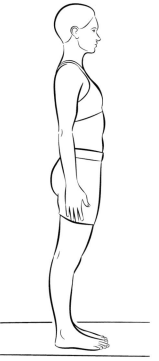

Once your arms return to your sides, you have completed one round of the sun salutation. As you begin again, change your leading lunge leg to step back with the left and continue alternating until you have completed an even number of your choice.

PART 2. THE EXERCISES
KYPHOSIS POSTURE

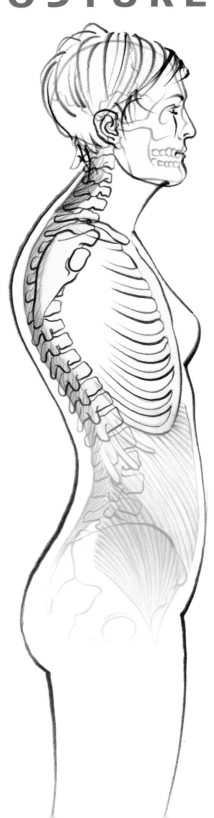

A kyphosis posture (which should technically be termed a hyperkyphosis posture) is where the thoracic spine exceeds the normal range of 35 degrees, meaning that the T1 vertebra effectively gets closer to the T12 vertebra.

In addition to the increase in thoracic curvature, there is normally a concomitant alteration of the lumbar curvature (hyper or hypolordosis), rotation of the pelvis (anterior or posterior), and flexion or extension in the hip joints.

As the thoracic spine increases its kyphosis, the scapulae will be abducted and the head will move forward (known as a forward head posture), causing the neck to extend in order to keep the eyes level with the horizon (which is essential for survival in the wild). The neck extensors will therefore be tight, and the neck flexors will be long and weak. With a kyphosis posture, there is amost always a tightening of the upper abdominal muscles and possibly also the pectoralis minor. There is also lengthening and weakening of the thoracic extensors and scapula adductors.

Physical causes

A kyphosis posture can be caused by a number of factors, all of which normally involve a form of faulty loading. This occurs when a muscle is loaded abnormally and can include trauma, overuse, or underuse. With faulty loading, tonic (postural) muscles tend to shorten and tighten. Phasic (mobilizer) muscles tend to lengthen and weaken.

The common causes of kyphosis posture are:

- Sitting in a slumped position for too long
- Working at a computer screen that is set up too low
- Carrying a poorly designed or poorly packed backpack
- Overarm sports, such as:
  - Tennis
  - Baseball
  - Swimming
  - Football
  - Cricket
- Cycling (in a hunched position)

- Too many abdominal crunch-type exercises
- Forward head posture
- Poor eyesight (therefore constantly leaning forward to look at things)
- Atlas subluxation (a misalignment of the first cervical vertebra)
- Being very tall and constantly needing to slump to speak to people
- Compensation for altered pelvic and lumbar spine position

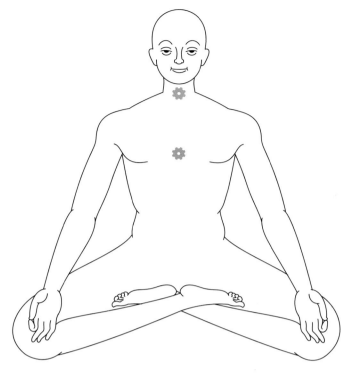

Emotional causes

There are many important psychosomatic relationships within the chest cavity. Emotions, thoughts, reactions, and expressions all get mixed up in the chest. The longer they are stored there, the more likely they are to create physical changes.

When looking at the structural changes of kyphosis, we have to take into consideration all the areas that are affected: shoulders, neck, upper back, and chest.

Forward hunched shoulders	Contracted chest	Forward head
Increased feelings of self-protection	Underdeveloped ability to be self-expressive and self-assertive	Encounter the world first with the head
Fear of being hurt	Feelings of insecurity	
Seeing ourselves as vulnerable	More passive than aggressive	
Emotional holding in the belly	More motivated by a chronic sense of fear and inferiority	

Possible related chakras

Chakra	Positive feelings cultivated	Location	Bija mantra
Heart chakra/4th—anahata	Compassion Unconditional love Forgiveness for oneself and others	The part of the vertebral column that relates to the heart/cardiac plexus	Yam
Throat chakra/5th—vishuddha	Truthful speech Honesty to oneself Freedom of self-expression	The neck region and the cervical part of the spinal column related to the throat/carotid plexus	Ham

The following pages show the sequence of exercises best practiced by those with a kyphotic posture.

LONGITUDINAL MOBILIZATIONS

Benefits
· Gravity helps stretch the ligaments in the front your spine, helping restore its natural curves.

· Take a foam roller or two rolled yoga mats and sit down on them. Slowly lower yourself so that the entire length of your spine and head rest on the roller. If you find that your head is tilted back and your chin is lifted, place a small rolled-up towel under the back of your head to keep the back of your neck lengthened.
· Keep your legs bent with your feet flat on the floor, aligning your knees with your hips.

· Take your arms up to shoulder height and bend your elbows to a 90 degree angle—at this point your fingers should be pointing upward—then gently lower the back of your hands to the floor. Try to keep the front of your rib cage down.
· Practice with a complete breath while relaxing on the roller (see page 72 for complete breath instructions). Stay in this position for at least five minutes, maintaining a connection with your breath.
· When finished, gently roll to the side and lie flat on the floor for a few moments, allowing the spine to settle.

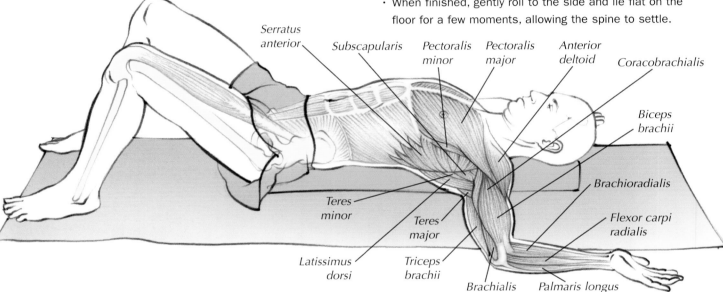

Serratus anterior · Subscapularis · Pectoralis minor · Pectoralis major · Anterior deltoid · Coracobrachialis · Biceps brachii · Brachioradialis · Flexor carpi radialis · Palmaris longus · Brachialis · Triceps brachii · Teres major · Teres minor · Latissimus dorsi

ANALYSIS OF MOVEMENT	REGION	JOINT MOVEMENT	MOBILIZED SECTION
Joint 1	Thoracic	Neutral spine	T4–T8

ANALYSIS OF MOVEMENT	JOINTS	JOINT MOVEMENT	MUSCLES ACTIVE	MUSCLES STRETCHED
Joint 1	Shoulder	Horizontal abduction, external rotation	Deltoid (posterior fibers), infraspinatus, teres minor	Pectotalis major, deltoid (anterior fibers), latissimus dorsi, teres major, subscapularis
Joint 2	Scapula	Downward rotation, adduction	Rhomboid major and minor, levator scapula, trapezius (middle fibers)	Trapezius (upper and lower fibers), serratus anterior, pectoralis minor
Joint 3	Elbow	Flexion	Biceps brachii, brachialis, brachioradilis, flexor carpi radialis, palmaris longus	

HORIZONTAL MOBILIZATIONS

- Place a rolled yoga mat or a 3–4-in. (8–10-cm) foam roller perpendicular to your spine. It is best to start with it just below your shoulder blades.
- Cradle your neck in your hands. Do not cradle your head.
- Slowly lower yourself down, with your neck supported, on an exhalation. Allow yourself to drop backward, going as far as is comfortable, draw your navel to your spine, and tilt the lower back to the floor.
- Stay in this position for three to five seconds, then come up. Repeat this a further three to five times.
- Slowly move up the spine, mobilizing each vertebra in the thoracic spine.

Benefits

- This is exceptionally effective for mobilizing each of the thoracic vertebra, but care must be taken—if you have arthritis or any spinal pathology, it should not be done.

- After completion, gently roll to the side to come off the roller/mat and lie flat on the floor to settle the spine.

If you feel discomfort in the spine after this, it is likely that you have done too much. You may need to reduce the time you stay in the position or reduce the repetitions.

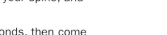 *Starting position*

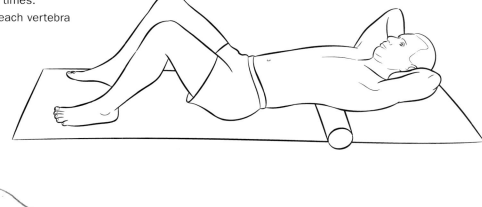

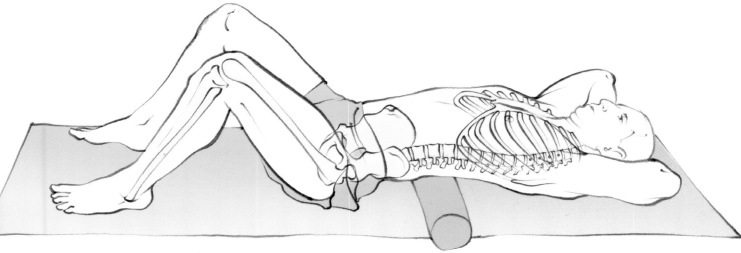

ANALYSIS OF MOVEMENT	REGION	JOINT MOVEMENT	JOINTS
Joint 1	Thoracic	Down: extension Up: flexion	T7–T3

MOVING CATS: MARJARIASANA

Benefits
- This awakens and warms the thoracic and lumbar spine to flexion and extension and the pelvis to anterior and posterior tilting. This is an ideal posture to do first thing in the morning.

- Go onto all fours, hands directly under your shoulders and knees under your hips.
- Keep the back of your neck in line with your spine.
- Breathe in deeply, then as you exhale, draw the navel to the spine and curl your spine upward, tilting your tailbone down and under. Drop your head, drawing your chin to your chest.
- Slightly contract the buttocks to assist this action.
- Press through your hands and lift your armpits from the floor, rounding your upper back to the ceiling.
- As you inhale, release the buttocks and reverse the tilt in your pelvis, allowing the tailbone to raise upward, creating a concave arch in your lumbar spine.
- Continue pressing through your hands as your chest lifts away from the floor. Try to allow the shoulder blades to sink down your back to the sacrum. Feel yourself lifting out of your shoulders.
- Allow your head to follow this movement, taking your gaze to the floor or to a point in front of you, and maintain the length in the back of your neck.
- Repeat this movement with your breath eight to ten times.

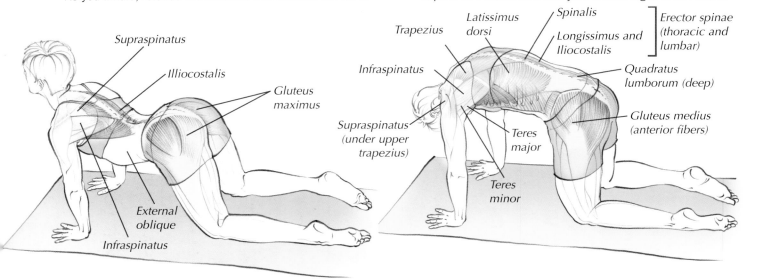

ANALYSIS OF MOVEMENT	JOINTS	JOINT MOVEMENT	MUSCLES ACTIVE
Joint 1	Scapula	UM: adduction and depression DM: abduction	UM: trapezius, latissimus dorsi DM: serratus anterior, pectoralis minor
Joint 2	Spine	UM: extension DM: flexion	UM: illiocostalis lumbar, thoracic, and cervicis, interspinalis cervicis and lumborum, spinalis, multifidi, semispinalis capitus, cervicis, and thoracis DM: internal and external obliques, transverse abdominus rectus, abdominus
Joint 3	Hip	UM: flexion DM: extension	UM: psoas major and minor, illiacus, anterior fibers, gluteus medius DM: gluteus maximus

(UM = upward movement; DM = downward movement)

SHOULDER OPENER 1

Benefits

· This is an effective anterior shoulder and chest opener, releasing tension and holding patterns in the chest area. It helps to improve flexibility of the accessory respiratory muscles.

· Sit in a comfortable position, in which you can maintain an erect spine. Take hold of a strap with your arms straight.

· As you inhale, slowly lift your arms upward, keeping them straight.

· As you exhale, slowly lower your arms down behind you. As you lower them, keep your lower rib cage from lifting upward.

· Have your hands wide enough apart to allow your arms to stay straight, keeping your gaze forward.

· Inhale and bring the arms back to vertical, then exhale to come back to the starting position.

· Try to keep the movement smooth and stretch outward from the shoulders as you make the circle.

· Repeat this six to eight times. Your breath should dictate the speed of the movement, so try to keep your breathing smooth, even, and slow.

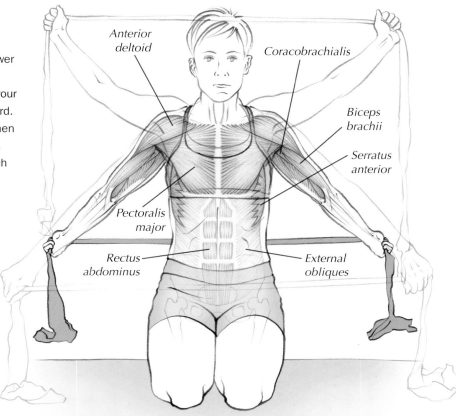

ANALYSIS OF MOVEMENT	JOINTS	JOINT MOVEMENT	MUSCLES ACTIVE	MUSCLES STRETCHED
Joint 1	Shoulder	UM: flexion DM: extension, external rotation	UM: anterior deltoid (upper fibers), pectoralis major, biceps brachii, coracobracialis DM: infraspinatus, teres minor, posterior deltoid, trapezius, rhomboids	DM: pectoralis major, anterior deltoid, biceps brachii, coracobrachialis, serratus anterior
Joint 2	Scapula	UM: upward rotation, abduction DM: downward rotation, adduction	UM: trapezius (upper and lower fibers), serratus anterior, pectoralis minor DM: rhomboid major and minor, levator scapula	UM: rhomboid major and minor, levator scapula DM: trapezius (upper and lower fibers) serratus anterior, pectoralis minor
Joint 3	Spine		Rectus abdominus, internal and external obliques, transverse abdominus	

(UM = upward movement; DM = downward movement)

SHOULDER OPENER 2

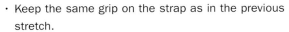

- Keep the same grip on the strap as in the previous stretch.
- Inhale, making your arms vertical. With your arms straight, as you exhale, take them back to the point where you feel the strongest stretch.
- Stay in this position for between one and two minutes. Keep the breath smooth and even.
- Engage your abdomen to draw your front ribs down, still maintaining a lift in your upper chest.

Benefits
- This is an effective anterior shoulder and chest opener, releasing tension and holding patterns in the chest area. It helps improve flexibility of the accessory respiratory muscles.

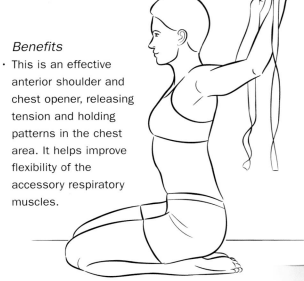

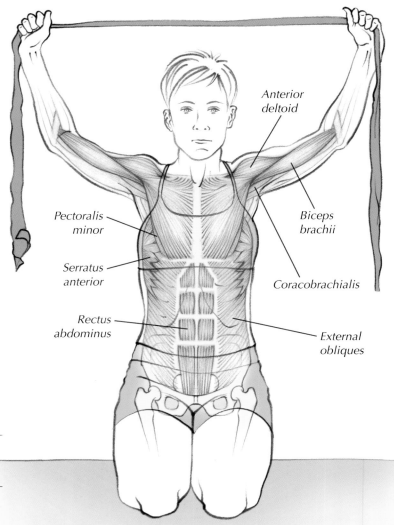

ANALYSIS OF MOVEMENT	JOINTS	JOINT MOVEMENT	MUSCLES ACTIVE	MUSCLES STRETCHED
Joint 1	Scapula	Downward rotation, adduction	Rhomboid major and minor, levator scapula	Trapezius (upper and lower fibers), serratus anterior, pectoralis minor
Joint 2	Shoulder	Extension, external rotation	Infraspinatus, teres minor, posterior deltoid, trapezius, rhomboids	Pectoralis major, anterior deltoid, biceps brachii, coracobracialis, serratus anterior
Joint 3	Spine	Stabilizing	Rectus abdominus, external and internal obliques, transverse abdominus	

SHOULDER OPENER 3

- Extend your right arm vertically, then bend your elbow and drop your hand between your shoulder blades.
- With your left hand, take hold of the top of your right elbow. Gently try to draw the elbow behind your head.
- Keep the abdomen firm and the front ribs low.
- Hold for several breaths, then repeat on the other side.
- Return to elevating the right arm to the beginning position and, while holding the arm here, take the left arm behind your back so the palm is facing away from you.
- Start to gently edge your left hand up toward your right hand. Do this gradually, allowing the shoulder to get used to this movement.
- If you can clasp your hands, then gently draw the elbows to the midline of your body and allow your elbows to move backward slightly from your body.
- Keep your abdomen firm and your front ribs low.
- Remain in the pose for between one and three minutes, maintaining an even breath.

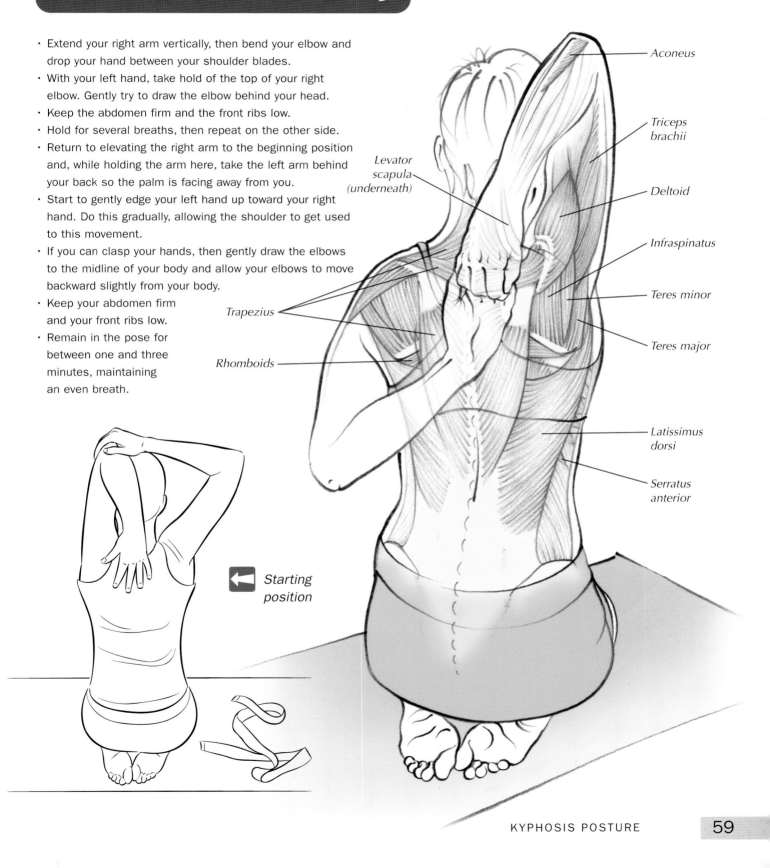

Aconeus

Triceps brachii

Deltoid

Infraspinatus

Teres minor

Teres major

Latissimus dorsi

Serratus anterior

Levator scapula (underneath)

Trapezius

Rhomboids

Starting position

SHOULDER OPENER 3

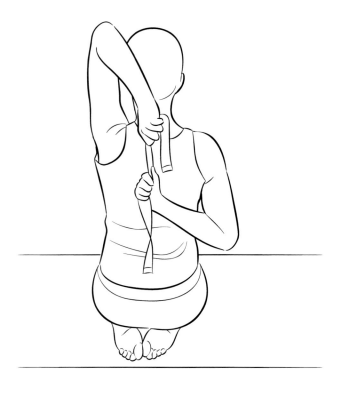

> *Modification*
> · If you are unable to clasp your hands, then place a strap or belt between your hands and after a while gently move your hands closer together.

Benefits
· Effective in releasing tension in the upper back and shoulders and will help increase rotation in the shoulder joint. Care must be taken not to overstretch and cause injury to the rotator cuff.

ANALYSIS OF MOVEMENT	JOINTS	JOINT MOVEMENT	MUSCLES ACTIVE	MUSCLES STRETCHED
Joint 1	Scapula	UA: upward rotation, abduction LA: downward rotation, adduction	UM: trapezius (upper and lower fibers), serratus anterior, pectoralis minor DM: rhomboid major and minor, levator scapula	UM: rhomboid major and minor, levator scapula DM: trapezius (upper and lower fibers), serratus anterior, pectoralis minor
Joint 2	Shoulder	UA: flexion, external rotation LA: extension, internal rotation	UA: deltoid, pectoralis major (upper fibers), biceps brachii, coracobrachialis, teres minor, infraspinatus LA: posterior and anterior deltoid, latissimus dorsi, teres major, infraspinatus, teres minor, pectoralis major, triceps brachii (long head), subscapularis	UA: triceps brachii (long head), anconeus, latissimus dorsi, teres minor, infraspinatus, teres major LA: rear deltoid, infraspinatus, teres minor
Joint 3	Elbow	UA: flexion, supination LA: flexion, pronation	UA: biceps brachii, brachialis, brachioradialis, flexor carpi radialis, palmaris longus, supinator LA: biceps brachii, brachialis, brachioradialis, flexor carpi radialis, palmaris longus, pronator teres, pronator quadratus	
Joint 4	Spine	Stabilization	Rectus abdominus, external and internal obliques, transverse abdominus	

(UA = upper arm; LA = lower arm; UM = upward movement; DM = downward movement)

SHOULDER OPENER 4

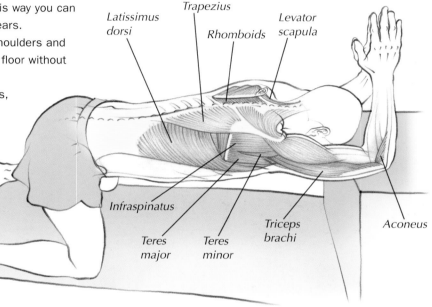

- Place the back of a chair against a wall with the seat facing you.
- Place your elbows shoulder-width apart on the edge of the chair and bring your hands into a "praying" position.
- Start to walk your knees back until they are directly underneath your hips and your spine is lengthened. Allow your forehead to rest on the edge of the chair.
- Keep the navel drawn in to the spine with the front ribs drawing away from your elbows. Try to keep your weight toward the outside edges of your elbows—this way you can keep space between the shoulders and the ears.
- Direct your breath into the upper back and shoulders and gradually allow the upper back to sink to the floor without arching your lower back.
- Remain here for at least two to three minutes, focusing on an even breath.

Benefits
- Effective in reversing the imbalance of excessive internal rotation of the arm. Also increases flexibility in the shoulders, thereby creating space to be able to hold the shoulders back. Improves flexibility of the accessory muscles of respiration.

Faulty alignment
- To make this stretch effective, your lumbar spine should not be arched. Note that you are engaging the abdominals in order to prevent this from happening.

Latissimus dorsi

Trapezius

Rhomboids

Levator scapula

Infraspinatus

Teres major

Teres minor

Triceps brachi

Aconeus

ANALYSIS OF MOVEMENT	JOINTS	JOINT MOVEMENT	MUSCLES ACTIVE	MUSCLES STRETCHED
Joint 1	Scapula	Upward rotation, abduction	Trapezius (upper and lower fibers), serratus anterior, pectoralis minor	Rhomboid major and minor, levator scapula
Joint 2	Shoulder	Flexion, external rotation	Deltoid, pectoralis major (upper fibers), biceps brachii, coracobrachialis, teres minor, infraspinatus	Triceps brachii (long head), anconeus, latissimus dorsi, teres minor, infraspinatus, teres major
Joint 3	Elbow	UA: flexion, pronation	Biceps brachii, brachialis, brachioradialis, flexor carpi radialis, palmaris longus, pronator teres, pronator quadratus	
Joint 4	Spine	Stabilization	Rectus abdominus, external and internal obliques, transverse abdominus	

(UA = upper arm)

SEATED TWIST: ARDHA MATSYENDRASANA

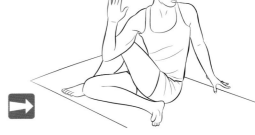

Front view

- Bend both legs, then lower your left knee down to the ground and place your heel to the outside of your right hip. Try to bring your left knee toward the midline of your body. Cross your right leg over the outside of the left knee so your foot is nestled into it. Keep your big toe grounded to the floor.
- Hold onto your right shin with both hands and pivot yourself forward onto the front of your buttock bones.
- Inhale, broadening and lifting your rib cage. Lift your right arm up and then backward, placing it on the floor in line with your sacrum, and exhale.
- Inhale and lift your left arm upward, then take your upper arm to the outside of your right knee, bending your elbow to 90 degrees so that your fingers are pointing upward.
- Exhale and lightly press the upper arm into the outside of the knee to create stability and the ability to lengthen the spine.

- Slowly turn your head back to look over your right shoulder, keeping your shoulders relaxed and your spine extended. Keep your gaze on the horizon and not on the floor.
- Maintain a smooth, even breath for between two to three minutes. Try to direct your breathing into the abdomen, keeping the chest relaxed.

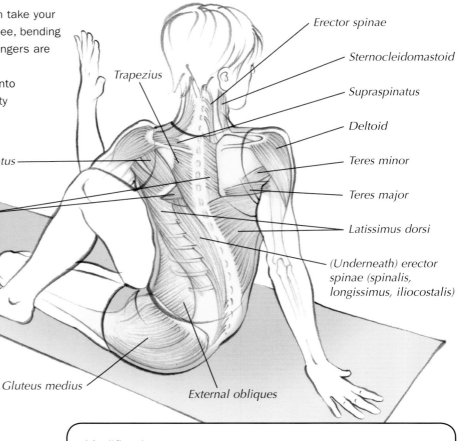

Trapezius

Erector spinae

Sternocleidomastoid

Supraspinatus

Deltoid

Infraspinatus

Teres minor

Teres major

Rhomboids

Latissimus dorsi

(Underneath) erector spinae (spinalis, longissimus, iliocostalis)

Gluteus medius

External obliques

Modification
- Start with the left leg straight and extend through the left heel as if pushing against a wall.
- Bend the right leg and place the right foot on the outside of your left thigh, grounding the sole of the foot and the big toe.
- Continue as with the full twist.

Benefits

· Effective in improving the rotation deep within the spine, which is necessary for healthy spinal mobility. Also stimulates the circulation and function of the internal organs and can assist in the elimination of toxins stored in the muscles and organ tissues.

ANALYSIS OF MOVEMENT	JOINTS	JOINT MOVEMENT	MUSCLES ACTIVE	MUSCLES STRETCHED
Joint 1	Elbow	FA: flexion BA: extension	FA: biceps brachii, brachialis, brachioradialis, flexor carpi radialis, palmaris longus BA: triceps brachii, anconeus	
Joint 2	Wrist	FA: neutral BA: extension		BA: flexor carpi radialis, flexor carpi ulnaris, palmaris longus, flexor digitorum superficialis, flexor digitorum profundus
Joint 3	Shoulder	FA: flexion moving toward extension, abduction, external rotation BA: external rotation, extension	FA: deltoid, pectoralis major (upper fibers), biceps brachii, coracobrachialis, deltoid, latissimus dorsi, teres major, infraspinatus, teres minor, pectoralis major, triceps brachii (long head), subscapularis, supraspinatus BA: deltoid, latissimus dorsi, teres major, infraspinatus, teres minor, pectoralis major, triceps brachii (long head)	BA: possibly pectoralis major, anterior deltoid
Joint 4	Scapula	FA: neutral BA: neutral	FA: rhomboids BA: rhomboids	
Joint 5	Spine	Spinal rotation toward top leg, neutral extension	TLS: internal obliques, erector spinae, splenius capitis BLS: external obliques, rotatores, multifidi, sternocleidomastoid, spinalis, longissimus, illiocostalis	TLS: external obliques, rotatores, multifidus, sternocleidomastoid BLS: internal obliques, erector spinae, splenius capitis, latissimus dorsi
Joint 6	Hip	TL: flexion, adduction, internal rotation BL: hip flexion, adduction, external rotation	TL: rectus femoris, adductor magnus, longus, and brevis, pectineus, gracilis, psoas major, illiacus, gluteus medius, gluteus minimus, semitendinosus, semimembranosus BL: rectus femoris, adductor magnus, longus, and brevis, pectineus, gracilis, psoas major, illiacus, biceps femoris, gluteus maximus, gluteus medius (posterior fibers), sartorius, piriformis, quadratus femoris, obturator internus and externus, gemellus superior and inferior	TL: piriformis, gemelli superior and inferior, obturator internus and externus, quadratus femoris, gluteus maximus, gluteus medius, gluteus minimus BL: piriformis, gluteus medius, gluteus minimus
Joint 7	Knee	Flexion	Biceps femoris, semitendinosus, semimembranosus, gracilis, sartorius, gastrocnemius, popliteus	

(FA = front arm; BA = back arm; TLS = top leg side; BLS = bottom leg side; TL = top leg; BL = bottom leg)

LOCUST POSE 1: SHALABASANA

- Lie face-down, straighten your legs, and press the tops of your feet lightly into the floor; your knees should lift.
- Place your arms alongside your body, with your palms to the floor, and rest your forehead on the floor.
- Draw the navel toward the spine, connecting with your core.
- Inhale slowly, then lift the chest, shoulders, hands, and head from the floor. Turn your hands out so that your palms are facing away from your body. Keep the back of your neck long and your gaze to the floor—resist the urge to jut your chin forward and look up.

Modification
- Keep your palms on the floor and lift your head, chest, and forehead. Keep the spine lengthened by extending the crown of the head forward and directing your gaze to the floor, chin slightly drawn back toward the throat.

- Keep the length within the spine by allowing the crown of the head to keep moving forward, away from the sacrum.
- Maintain a smooth, even breath. Hold the pose for up to four minutes—this will dramatically increase the strength in the back musculature.

Benefits
- Strengthens both the lower back muscles and the upper back. Can help poor digestion.

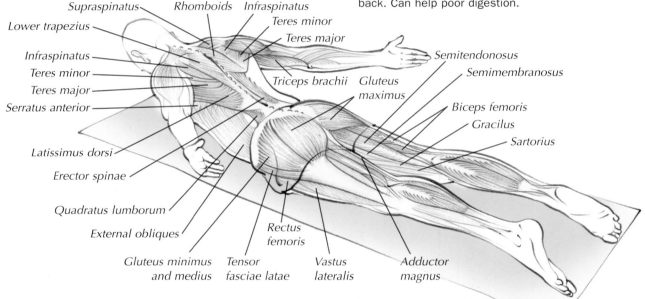

Supraspinatus — Rhomboids — Infraspinatus — Teres minor — Teres major — Lower trapezius — Infraspinatus — Teres minor — Teres major — Serratus anterior — Triceps brachii — Gluteus maximus — Semitendonosus — Semimembranosus — Biceps femoris — Gracilus — Sartorius — Latissimus dorsi — Erector spinae — Quadratus lumborum — External obliques — Rectus femoris — Gluteus minimus and medius — Tensor fasciae latae — Vastus lateralis — Adductor magnus

ANALYSIS OF MOVEMENT	JOINTS	JOINT MOVEMENT	MUSCLES ACTIVE
Joint 1	Scapula	Downward rotation, adduction	Rhomboid major and minor, levator scapula
Joint 2	Shoulder	Extension, external rotation	Posterior deltoid, latissimus dorsi, teres major, subscapularis, pectoralis major, teres minor, infraspinatus, triceps brachii (long head)
Joint 3	Spine	Extension	Spinalis, longissimus, ilicostalis, multifidi, rotatores, semispinalis capitis, intertransversarii, interspinalis
Joint 4	Hip	Extension, internal rotation, adduction	Biceps femoris, semitendinosus, semimembranosus, gluteus maximus, gluteus medius (anterior fibers), adductor magnus, longus and brevis, gracilis, pectineus, tensor fasciae latae
Joint 5	Knee	Extension	Rectus femoris, vastus lateralis, medialis, and intermedius

BACK BRIDGE: SETU BANDASANA

- Lay flat on the floor, then bring your heels toward your buttocks, in line with your sitting bones.
- Place your arms by your sides, palms down.
- On your exhalation, press your feet and arms firmly to the floor and gradually lift your hips from the floor.
- Lift your hips as high as is comfortable for your lower back; the knees should stay in line with the hips. Tilt the pubic bone toward you, allowing your buttocks to move toward your legs.

- After a few breaths, bring the backs of your arms closer together and interlace your fingers. Press the upper arms to the floor, encouraging the sternum to lift. Lift the hips a little higher if you feel that you can.
- The navel should be lightly drawn to the spine, protecting the lower back.
- Maintain an even breath, holding the pose for between two and three minutes.

Benefits
- Increases flexibility in the anterior shoulders and chest, improves breathing patterns, and strengthens the back.

Biceps femoris Semitendinosus

Semimembranosus

External and internal obliques Tensor fasciae latae

Latissimus dorsi

Serratus anterior

Pectoralis major

Pectoralis minor

Gluteus maximus

Gluteus medius

Deltoid Triceps brachii

Spinalis, longissimus, iliocostalis

BACK BRIDGE: SETU BANDASANA

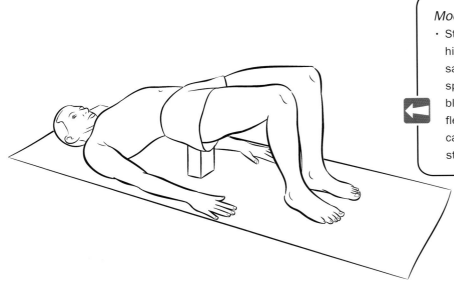

Modification
- Starting in the same position, as you lift your hips, place a foam block underneath the sacrum—it should not rest on the lumbar spine. You can change the direction of the block you are resting on depending on how flexible you are. While in this position, you can rest the hips completely on the block, still keeping the feet and arms active.

ANALYSIS OF MOVEMENT	JOINTS	JOINT MOVEMENT	MUSCLES ACTIVE	MUSCLES STRETCHED
Joint 1	Scapula	Downward rotation, adduction	Rhomboid major and minor, levator scapula	Trapezius (upper and lower fibers), serratus anterior, pectoralis minor
Joint 2	Shoulder	Extension, external rotation, adduction	Posterior deltoid, latissimus dorsi, teres major, subscapularis, pectoralis major, teres minor, infraspinatus, triceps brachii (long head), coracobrachialis	Pectoralis major
Joint 3	Elbow	Extension, supination	Triceps brachii, aconeus, biceps brachii, supinator, brachioradialis	
Joint 4	Spine	Extension	Spinalis, longissimus, ilicostalis, multifidi, rotatores, semispinalis capitis, intertransversarii, interspinalis	Psoas minor, rectus abdominus, external and internal obliques
Joint 5	Hip	Extension, internal rotation, adduction	Biceps femoris, semitendinosus, semimembranosus, gluteus maximus, gluteus medius (posterior fibers), adductor magnus, longus, and brevis, gracilis, pectineus, tensor fasciae latae	Rectus femoris, psoas major, iliacus
Joint 6	Knee	Extension	Rectus femoris, vastus lateralis, medialis, and intermedius	
Joint 7	Ankle	Dorsiflexion	Tibialis anterior, extensor digitorum longus, extensor hallucis longus	

CAMEL POSE: USTRASANA

Benefits
- Effective in stretching the chest area and releasing tension in the abdominal muscles and internal organs. Improves breathing patterns.

- Come into an upright kneeling position. Align your hips over your knees and keep your ankles in line with your knees, with your feet straight back.
- Press your shins, knees, and feet to the floor and extend your spine and crown of your head to the ceiling. Squeeze your legs together without moving them and keep your thighs vertical.
- Lift your chest and thoracic spine, creating length in your lower back. Press your sacrum and tailbone down and firmly forward.
- Place your hands on your buttocks, fingertips down. Draw the inner elbows toward each other.
- Inhale, lifting the chest, and as you exhale, draw the navel to the spine and arch your back, moving your elbows back and down as your chest remains lifted. Keep the legs active and thighs vertical as you gently release your hands to your heels.

- Roll your shoulders back and push downward through your hands, lifting your chest. Focus on length in your spine as the sacrum and tailbone move forward.
- There should be no strain in the lower back. See the modifications for different stages of the asana.
- To come out of the pose, press firmly through your feet and rise up straight—try not to twist the spine. Lead upward with your chest and come back to kneeling.
- Focus on maintaining an even and smooth breath. If you find your breath becoming uneven, then come out of the pose. If you can maintain an even breath, hold the pose for up to three minutes.

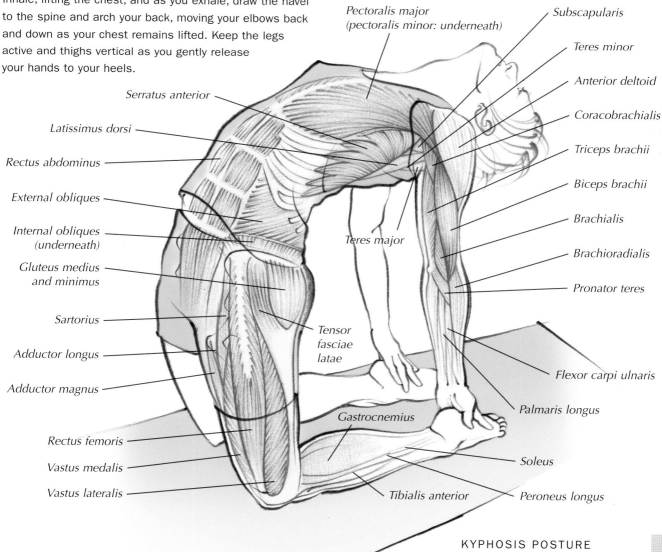

Serratus anterior

Latissimus dorsi

Rectus abdominus

External obliques

Internal obliques (underneath)

Gluteus medius and minimus

Sartorius

Adductor longus

Adductor magnus

Rectus femoris

Vastus medalis

Vastus lateralis

Pectoralis major (pectoralis minor: underneath)

Subscapularis

Teres minor

Anterior deltoid

Coracobrachialis

Triceps brachii

Biceps brachii

Brachialis

Brachioradialis

Pronator teres

Teres major

Tensor fasciae latae

Gastrocnemius

Tibialis anterior

Flexor carpi ulnaris

Palmaris longus

Soleus

Peroneus longus

CAMEL POSE: USTRASANA

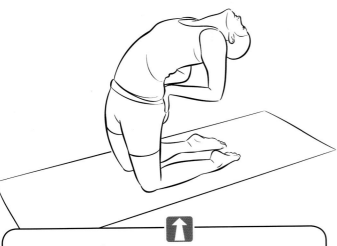

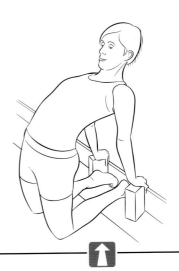

Modification 1
· Remain with your hands on your buttocks and focus on the activity of your legs. Keep the inner elbows pressing toward each other and down—this will encourage the chest to lift and open.

Modification 2
· Move close to a wall and place two blocks on either side of your outer heels. Follow the same sequence of points and allow the hands to move back onto the blocks. The back of your head should rest lightly on the wall; do not press through the head, just allow it to rest—this will help to support the neck.

ANALYSIS OF MOVEMENT	JOINTS	JOINT MOVEMENT	MUSCLES ACTIVE	MUSCLES STRETCHED
Joint 1	Scapula	Downward rotation, adduction	Rhomboid major and minor, levator scapula	Serratus anterior, pectoralis minor
Joint 2	Shoulder	Extension, external rotation, adduction	Posterior deltoid, latissimus dorsi, teres major, subscapularis, pectoralis major, teres minor, infraspinatus, triceps brachii (long head), coracobrachialis	Pectoralis major
Joint 3	Elbow	Extension, supination	Triceps brachii, aconeus, biceps brachii, supinator, brachioradialis	Coracobrachialis, biceps brachii
Joint 4	Spine	Extension	Spinalis, longissimus, ilicostalis, multifidi, rotatores, semispinalis capitis, intertransversarii, interspinalis	Psoas minor, rectus abdominus, external and internal obliques
Joint 5	Hip	Extension, internal rotation, adduction	Biceps femoris, semitendinosus, semimembranosus, gluteus maximus, gluteus medius (posterior fibers), adductor magnus, longus and brevis, gracilis, pectineus, tensor fasciae latae	Rectus femoris, psoas major, iliacus
Joint 6	Knee	Extension	Rectus femoris, vastus lateralis, medialis, and intermedius	
Joint 7	Ankle	Dorsiflexion	Tibialis anterior, extensor digitorum longus, extensor hallucis longus	

HALF SHOULDERSTAND: ARDHA SALAMBA SARVANGASANA

- Begin by lying on the floor, with your heels toward your bottom and your arms to your sides, palms down.
- Inhale, then as you exhale, press your hands into the floor and lift your hips off the floor, swinging your legs toward your head.
- Inhale, then as you exhale, bend your arms, bringing your forearms vertical. Bring your inner elbows as close together as possible, then slowly lower your hips into your hands.
- Press your upper arms into the floor and away from your shoulders, with your inner elbows pressing toward each other—this is very similar to camel pose.
- Try not to collapse the thoracic spine—keep it elevated. Straighten your legs and lift them to a comfortable height, pressing your inner thighs together and flexing your feet.
- Stay in the pose for two to three minutes with a smooth, even, diapraghmatic breath.
- To come out of the pose, bend your knees to your chest, release your arms to the floor palms down, then slowly lower your back to the floor. As your feet come to the floor, straighten one leg at a time.

Benefits
- A powerful soothing effect on the nervous system. It helps balance the endocrine glands and metabolic functions, improves circulation, and reduces fluid retention. Effective in improving respiratory patterns.

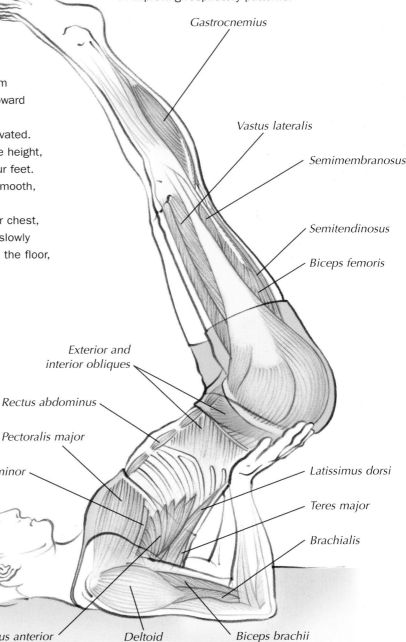

Starting position

Gastrocnemius

Vastus lateralis

Semimembranosus

Semitendinosus

Biceps femoris

Exterior and interior obliques

Rectus abdominus

Pectoralis major

Pectoralis minor

Latissimus dorsi

Teres major

Brachialis

Serratus anterior

Deltoid

Biceps brachii

HALF SHOULDERSTAND: ARDHA SALAMBA SARVANGASANA

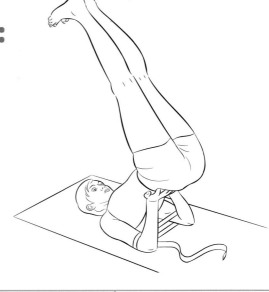

> *Modification*
> - Place a strap around one arm above the elbow, then when ready, lift your hips off the floor, swinging your legs toward your head. At this point, put your other arm into the strap. Bending both elbows, place your hands on your back.

ANALYSIS OF MOVEMENT	JOINTS	JOINT MOVEMENT	MUSCLES ACTIVE	MUSCLES STRETCHED
Joint 1	Scapula	Downward rotation, adduction	Rhomboid major and minor, levator scapula	Serratus anterior, pectoralis minor
Joint 2	Shoulder	External rotation, extension, adduction	Posterior deltoid, infraspinatus, teres minor, latissimus dorsi, teres major, pecotoralis major, triceps brachii (long head), coracobrachialis	Coracobrachialis, pectoralis major
Joint 3	Elbow	Flexion, forearm supination	Biceps brachii, brachialis, brachioradialis, flexor carpi radialis, palmaris longus, supinator	All muscles crossing the elbow joint will be stretched
Joint 4	Wrist	Extension	Extensor carpi radialis longus, extensor carpi radialis brevis, extensor carpi ulnaris	Flexor carpi radialis and ulnaris, palmaris longus, flexor digitorum superficialis
Joint 5	Spine: cervical, upper thoracic	Flexion	The neck flexors should not be active	Trapezius (upper fibers), levator scapula, splenius capitus, splenius cervicis, rectus capitis posterior major and minor, oblique capitis superior, semispinalis capitis, longissimus capitis and cervicis, iliocastalis cervicis
Joint 6	Spine: lower thoracic, lumbar	Extension	Spinalis, longissimus, ilicostalis, multifidi, rotatores, semispinalis capitis, intertransversarii, interspinalis, external and internal obliques, rectus abdominus, transverse abdominus working eccentrically	The musculature of the torso will be active
Joint 7	Hip	Flexion, adduction, internal rotation	Psoas minor	
Joint 8	Knee	Extension	Rectus femoris, vastus lateralis, vastus medialis	Gastronemius

CORPSE POSE: SAVASANA

"Sava" means corpse: this is a deep relaxation pose where the body is motionless, looking like a corpse. We spend most of our daily lives moving, rarely enjoying stillness; practicing this pose is a time to experience deep stillness and inner calm. Concentrate your mind on the subtle movements of your breath and the rise and fall of your abdomen. On each exhalation, have a sense of letting go of tension; allow the body to surrender to gravity. Try not to get caught in unnecessary thoughts. Just allow the body to be.

- Start on your back with your heels toward the sitting bones, then gently straighten one leg at a time. Stretch the legs away from you, draw the pubic bone toward you for a second, lengthening the lower back, then relax.
- Have the legs a little wider than hip-width apart. Straighten your arms away from your body, palms up, and relax your shoulders down away from your ears. Lengthen your head away from your shoulders
- Soften the skin of your face and let your jaw slightly part. Rest here for at least five to ten minutes.

- When you have finished, roll onto your right side, rest here for a few moments, and open your eyes. Gently bring yourself into a sitting position, becoming aware of your surroundings.
- If, during the pose, you find tension building in your neck, place a small blanket underneath your neck to help keep it lengthened. You may also place a blanket underneath your knees to take any stress out of the lower back. An eyemask can be used on the eyes, as this is effective in calming the nervous system.

Benefits
- "Lying upon one's back on the ground at full length like a corpse, removes fatigue caused by the other asana and induces calmness of mind" (S. Muktibodhananda, *Hatha Yoga Pradipika*). This posture gives the body time to relax and enjoy stillness. It has a calming effect on the nervous system.

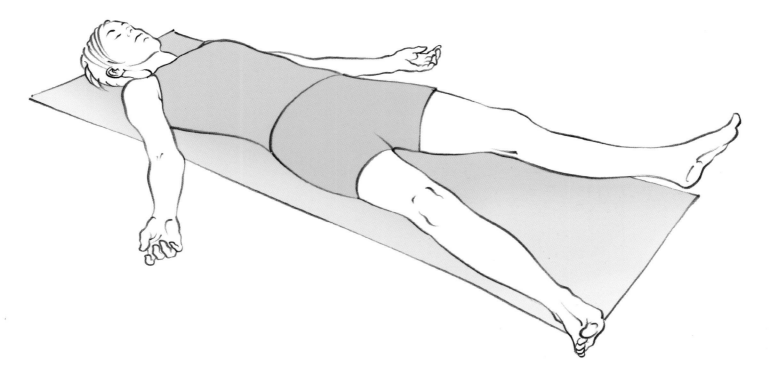

In a kyphotic posture, the thoracic spine has an increased convex curve. This will affect the placement of the rib cage, affecting the efficiency of your breathing pattern. For the lungs to expand fully, there must be flexibility in the intercostal muscles (which lie in between each of the ribs), the rib cage, and the spine. The following breathing practice will focus on stretching and mobilizing the thoracic cavity.

Complete breath practice

You will need a rolled up mat or a foam roller placed on the floor. Gently lower yourself down onto the roller or mat so that the entire length of your spine and head are resting on it. Bend your legs so that your feet are placed firmly on the floor and allow your arms to come to shoulder height, with the palms up.

Start to settle yourself. Allow the back of your shoulders and elbows to descend to the floor, feeling a light stretch across your upper chest. Soften your neck and the muscles of your face. Stay here for a few moments, bringing your mind and body together in union by focusing your attention with the subtle movements of your breath. Relax every muscle and joint in your body.

When you feel that your mind and body have settled, place both hands on your abdomen. Start to direct your breath into the lower abdomen. As you inhale, feel your abdomen lifting into your hands, and as you exhale, feel your abdomen falling toward your spine and away from your hands. Stay with this pattern for a few breaths. Then move your hands to the bottom of your rib cage, the heels of your hands resting on the outer rib cage and the fingers resting over the top. Start to direct your breath into your lower rib cage. Feel how the rib cage expands into your hands as you inhale and decreases in size as you exhale. Stay with this for a few moments, connecting with the movement.

Now move your hands to rest on your upper chest. Just for a few breaths, direct your inhalation and exhalation high up into the chest—do not do this for long. Allow your breath to return back to its natural pattern. Move one hand down to rest on your abdomen and leave the other hand resting on your chest. On your next inhalation, start the breath in the abdomen for the first third of the breath, feeling your bottom hand move. Then allow the breath to move into your lower rib cage for the second third of the inhalation. Then for the final third of the inhalation, feel your upper chest lift just a small amount into your top hand. Exhale smoothly and evenly. Continue to repeat this cycle with each inhalation, expanding the entire circumference of the torso and trying to become aware of the subtle movements to the front and back of the body.

Continue with this rhythm for five minutes. In the last few minutes of the practice, release your hands down to the floor and return your arms to shoulder height: this will stretch the chest muscles passively. Eventually you will be able to practice without the aid of your hands for direction. They can stay at shoulder height throughout the entire practice.

There will only be a small movement in the very top part of your upper chest—try not to force this movement mechanically as it will cause tension in the neck and shoulders. Throughout the entire practice, keep your face, neck, and shoulders relaxed.

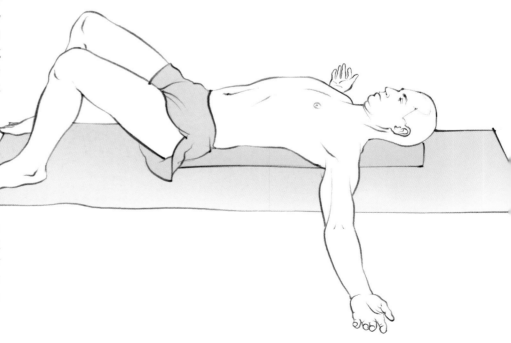

KYPHOSIS POSTURE

Mantras are an integral part of yogic meditation. When reciting a mantra either mentally or verbally, there are vibrational effects that are transformative both mentally and physically. An important factor is that when reciting the mantra, it should be fully impressed upon the mind, leaving no room for thoughts.

The "So Hum" meditation is known as the universal meditation or "mahamantra"—the greatest mantra. It relates directly to the sound of one's breath. As you listen intently to your breath, you will notice that as you inhale there is the sound "so," and as you exhale you will hear the sound "hum." Listening to these sounds is not the only beauty of this mantra: it has a more transformative effect on the individual consciousness. "So Hum" translates as "I am that" or "I am that I am." The mantra's aim is to bring union between individual consciousness and divine consciousness, to realize that all that you see is yourself; the observer is the observed.

The practice

Bring yourself into a comfortable seated position with your hands in jnana mudra (forefinger and thumb together, facing down to calm the mind). Start to bring your awareness to your body: scan the body, taking your mind to each of the following body parts. Start with your right thumb, moving then to your index finger, middle finger, ring finger, little finger, palm of your hand, top of your hand, wrist, forearm, elbow, upper arm, shoulder, right side of your chest, right shoulder blade, right side of your waist, side, back, right hip bone, right buttock, right thigh, right knee, right shin, calf, ankle, top of the foot, sole of the foot, right big toe, second toe, third toe, fourth toe, and little toe. Move your mind and focus on your left thumb, moving then to your index finger, middle finger, ring finger, little finger, palm of the hand, top of the hand, wrist, forearm, elbow, upper arm, shoulder, left side of the chest, left shoulder blade, left side of the waist, side, back, left hip bone, left buttock, right thigh, left knee, left shin, calf, ankle, top of the foot, sole of the foot, left big toe, second toe, third toe, fourth toe, and little toe. Then pause for a few moments and start to focus on your breathing.

Allow your entire body to relax. Feel the crown of your head lifting to the ceiling and your chin dropping slightly and moving back to the throat. Allow

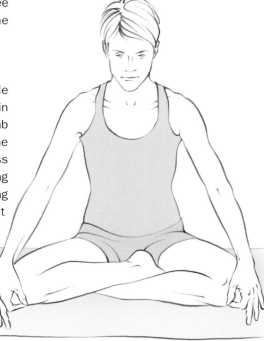

your breath to move evenly and smoothly through your nose and relax your abdomen.

Observe the rise and fall of your breath.

On your next inhalation, silently say "so" to yourself, allowing the word to last the length of the inhalation.

As you exhale, silently say "hum" to yourself, allowing the word to last the length of the exhalation.

Keep your focus on the sensation of your breath while silently repeating the two syllables of "so hum." Allow the breath to draw along the back of your throat and start to listen for the sounds that your breathing makes. Let your mind become absorbed in the sounds. If your attention starts to drift away to bodily sensations, sounds in your environment or internal chatter, then gently move your focus back to the breath and "so hum." This may happen a few times, but try not to become frustrated with your wandering attention, as this is all part of the journey. Just gently and lovingly return the mind to its focus.

If you are a beginner to seated meditation, then sit for as long as you feel comfortable. As you become more adept, set a timer for 10 to 30 minutes. As you come to the end of your practice, move your awareness away from your breath and the mantra and finally sit in silence. Contemplate within your heart space the essence of "I am that" and feel your connection to the supreme consciousness.

When you are ready, slowly open your eyes, become aware of your surroundings, stretch your body, then move forth with love and gratitude in your heart.

LORDOSIS POSTURE

A lordosis posture is where the lumbar spine exceeds the normal range of 35 degrees and the L1 vertebra effectively gets closer to the L5 vertebra. In addition to the increase in lumbar curvature, there is normally a concomitant anterior rotation of the pelvis and flexion of the hip joints.

The thoracic spine will compensate above it to maintain the center of gravity by increasing its kyphosis, which creates a forward head posture. As the thoracic spine increases its kyphosis, the scapulae will also be abducted. The knees will tend to hyperextend and the ankles will slightly plantarflex due to the backward angle of the leg, and the weight on the feet will move to the forefoot.

With a lordosis posture, there is almost always a tightening of the iliopsoas muscles and possibly also the rectus femoris and other hip flexors. The neck extensors are normally tight and the lumbar erector muscles are normally strong and may or may not be short. There is also lengthening and weakening of the external obliques, neck flexors, and thoracic extensors. The hamstrings tend to be elongated, but may or may not be weak. The lower abdominal muscles (rectus abdominis below the naval, as well as the external and internal obliques) tend to be weak.

Physical causes

A lordosis posture can be caused by a number of factors, all of which also involve a form of faulty loading.

It is generally believed that this posture begins with a tightening of the psoas muscle. The other muscle imbalances then occur in an attempt to maintain as much balance over the base of support as possible.

A tightening of the psoas muscle can be caused by:

- Sitting for long periods
- Sports such as:
  - Long-distance running
  - Cycling
  - Martial arts
  - Soccer
  - Gymnastics (could also create a lordosis due to the frequent and excessive lumbar extension required)
- Wearing high-heeled shoes
- Dancing
- Structural flat feet, although this is rare. Note also that all humans are born with flat feet. The arch in the foot

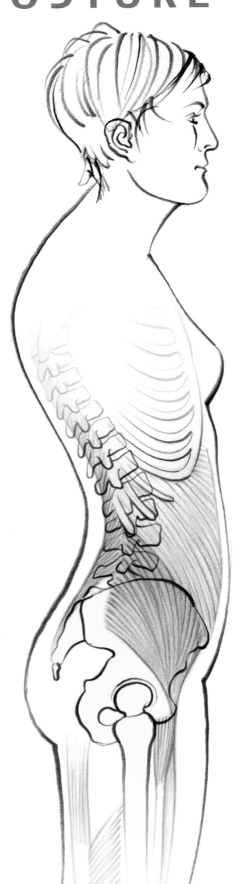

normally begins to develop shortly after a child begins to walk and finishes developing around the age of seven.

Emotional causes

There are many important psychosomatic relationships around the pelvis and abdominal area. The belly is known as the "feeling center of the bodymind" (K. Dychtwald, *Bodymind*). It is within the belly that our emotions and passions originate. You may have found yourself using terms such as "I have butterflies in my stomach" when approaching a challenge or "I feel sick to my stomach"during a confrontation. Blocked emotions and feelings that originate in the belly and are not fully expressed will become stressfully trapped within this area. The longer they are stored in the region, the more likely they are to create physical changes.

When looking at the structural changes of lordosis, we have to take into consideration all the areas that are affected. The pelvis is an obvious area of physical change. The upper body will also undergo changes due to the alignment of the pelvis.

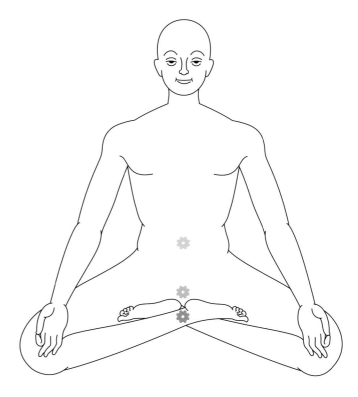

Anterior pelvic tilt	Rounded shoulders	Contracted chest
Heightening of sexual energy	Tendency to take on too many responsibilities	Underdeveloped ability to be self-expressive and self-assertive
A strong need for security	Feelings of being overburdened by life itself	More motivated by a chronic sense of fear and inferiority
Worries about the needs of others		Will be more passive than aggressive
Abundunce of internal feelings		Feelings of insecurity

Chakra	Positive feelings cultivated	Location	Bija mantra
Root chakra/1st—muladhara	Grounding Inner strength Stability	Perineum, below the genitals and above the anus, inside the coccyx; related to the pelvic plexus	Lam
Sacral chakra/ 2nd—svadhistahana	Self-love Worthy of love Acceptance of how perfect you are	Genital area, hypogastric plexus	Vam
Solar plexus chakra/ 3rd—manipura	Self-confidence Courage Fearless of life's challenges	The part of the vertebral column that relates to the navel; solar plexus	Ram

FORWARD BEND: UTTANASANA

Benefits
- This helps improve flexibility in the legs and lower back. It is said to relieve stomach pains and is also effective in calming the nervous system.

- Stand with your feet hip-width apart and evenly distribute your weight through the balls and heels of your feet.
- Your inner ankles should be vertical, not rolling inward or outward. Keep your kneecaps lifted and your thigh muscles contracted.
- Elongate your spine outward from the crown of your head and draw your chin slightly in toward your throat, feeling the back of your neck extend.
- Keep your armpits lifted but your shoulders moving down.
- Inhale and extend to the ceiling with your chest and arms. As you exhale, pivot forward at your hips, lifting your sitting bones as you move.
- Take your hands to rest just below your knees, lengthen your spine, and lift your sitting bones.
- Stretch forward from the crown of your head. On your next exhalation, shift your hands to your ankles, holding behind the ankles, thumbs pointing to the floor and elbows bent backward. Roll your thighs in and lift your shoulders away from the floor. Maintain length in your spine and space under your ribs. If you feel able to take your hands down to lie flat on the floor, do so, being very careful not to go farther than is comfortable.
- It is important to keep the spine straight. If your hamstrings are especially tight, bend your knees and gradually work with the breath to straighten them. It is important not to hyperextend the knees—keep the knees slightly bent if this happens.
- Remain in the pose for up to three minutes, with an even breath.

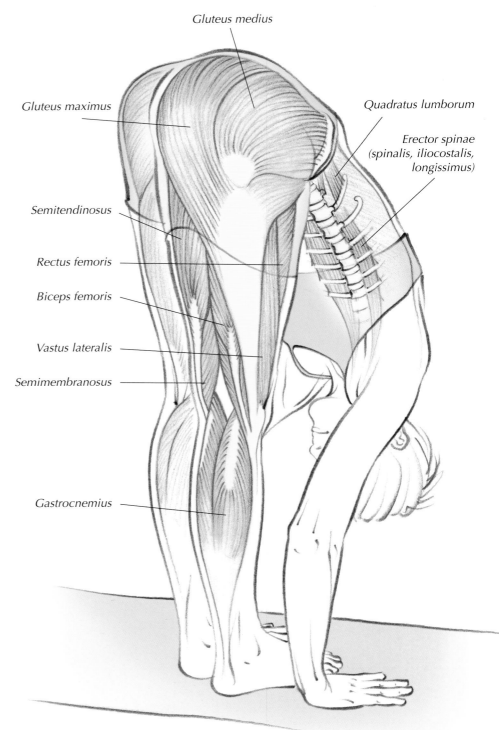

Gluteus medius

Gluteus maximus

Quadratus lumborum

Erector spinae
(spinalis, iliocostalis, longissimus)

Semitendinosus

Rectus femoris

Biceps femoris

Vastus lateralis

Semimembranosus

Gastrocnemius

> **Note:**
> - In this pose, gravity should draw the torso down. When there is extreme tightness in the hamstrings, people tend to pull themselves down, which can create tension in the psoas muscles and abdominals. It is better to keep the knees bent and to just use the hands holding the ankles as an anchor. In the following breakdown of muscles the arms have been left out.

> **Modification 1**
> - Keep your knees bent if you find that there is too much strain on your hamstrings.

> **Modification 2**
> - Place two blocks on the floor on either side of your feet. Follow the same steps as before, placing your hands on the blocks instead of on the floor or your ankles. You can also use a chair.

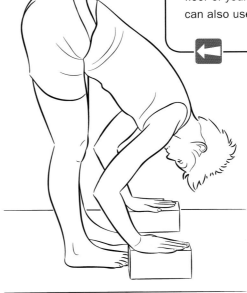

ANALYSIS OF MOVEMENT	JOINTS	JOINT MOVEMENT	MUSCLES ACTIVE	MUSCLES STRETCHED
Joint 1	Scapula	Downward rotation, adduction	Rhomboid major, rhomboid minor, levator scapula, trapezius (middle fibers)	Possibly pectoralis minor
Joint 2	Spine	Flexion		Spinalis, longissimus, ilicostalis, multifidi, rotatores, semispinalis capitis, intertransversarii, quadratus lumborum, interspinalis
Joint 3	Hip	Flexion		Biceps femoris, semitendinosus, semimembranosus, gluteus maximus, gluteus medius (posterior fibers), adductor magnus
Joint 4	Knee	Extension	Vastus medialis, vastus lateralis, rectus femoris	Gastrocnemius

YOGIC SQUAT: UPAVESANA

Front view →

- Stand with your feet a little wider than hip-width apart. Turn your feet out about 30 degrees and inhale. As you exhale, slowly bend your knees deeply, lowering yourself as far down as you can. Keep a strong abdominal connection by drawing in your navel.
- Reach your arms in front of your knees and then press your upper arms against the front of your knees. As you do this, draw your chest forward between your arms, extending the upper spine.
- Keep a strong lift in the pelvic floor, perineum, and transversus abdominus.
- Maintain a steady breath and remain in the pose for up to two minutes.

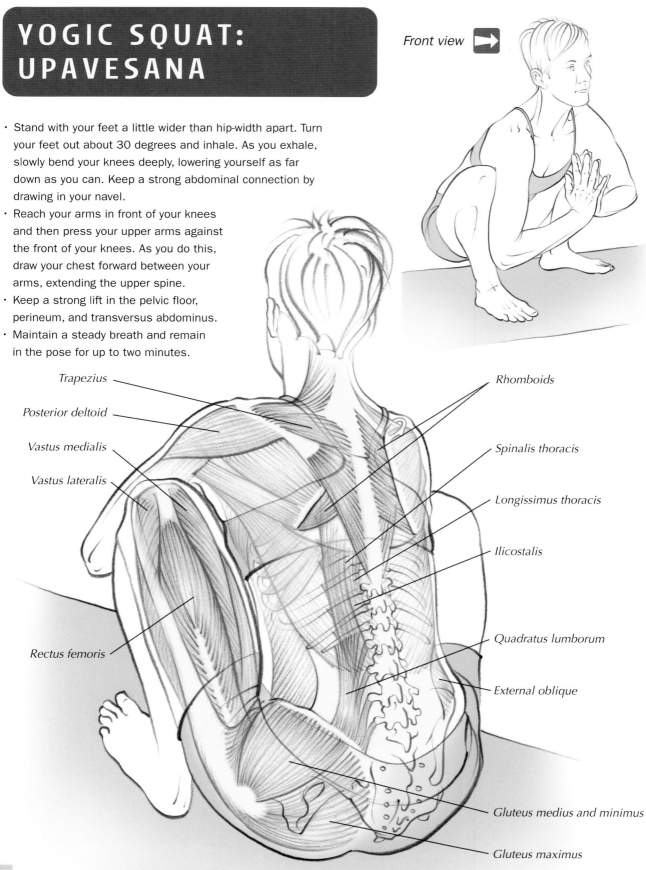

Trapezius

Posterior deltoid

Vastus medialis

Vastus lateralis

Rectus femoris

Rhomboids

Spinalis thoracis

Longissimus thoracis

Ilicostalis

Quadratus lumborum

External oblique

Gluteus medius and minimus

Gluteus maximus

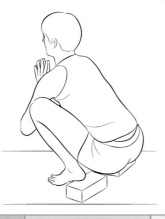

Benefits
· Increases flexibility and strength in the ankles and feet, aids digestion, and increases flexion in the spine.

Modification
· Place blocks or a rolled-up blanket underneath your heels before you squat. Make sure that you don't become reliant on this prop as it will prevent the achilles tendon and soleus from stretching, which improves the range of motion in your ankles.

ANALYSIS OF MOVEMENT	JOINTS	JOINT MOVEMENT	MUSCLES ACTIVE	MUSCLES STRETCHED
Joint 1	Spine: cervical, thoracic	Extension	Spinalis, longissimus, ilicostalis, multifidi, rotatores, semispinalis capitis, intertransversarii, interspinalis	
Joint 2	Spine: lumbar	Flexion	Rectus abdominus, external and internal obliques	Spinalis (lower fibers), longissimus, ilicostalis, multifidi, rotatores, semispinalis capitis, intertransversarii, quadratus lumborum, interspinalis
Joint 3	Scapula	Adduction	Trapezius (middle fibers), rhomboid major and minor	
Joint 4	Shoulder	External rotation, adduction, extension	Posterior deltoid, infraspinatus, teres minor, latissimus dorsi, teres major, pecotoralis major, triceps brachii (long head), coracobrachialis	
Joint 5	Elbow	Flexion, pronation	Biceps brachii, brachialis, brachioradialis, flexor carpi radialis, palmaris longus, pronator teres, pronator quadratus	
Joint 6	Wrist	Extension	Extensor carpi radialis longus, extensor carpi radialis brevis, extensor carpi ulnaris	
Joint 7	Hip	Flexion, abduction	Rectus femoris, gluteus medius (anterior fibers), gluteus minimus, tensor fasciae latae, sartorius, psoas major, iliacus, gluteus maximus	Adductor longus, adductor brevis
Joint 8	Knee	Flexion	Biceps femoris, semitendinosus, semimembranosus, gracilis, sartorius, gastrocnemius, popliteus	
Joint 9	Ankle	Dorsiflexion	Tibialis anterior, extensor digitorum longus, extensor hallucis longus	Gastrocnemius, soleus, plantaris, peroneus longus, peroneus brevis

FRONT THIGH STRETCH

- Come into an upright kneeling position, then take one leg forward so that both legs are at a 90 degree angle. Allow the front knee to move over the toes slightly. Inhale.
- As you exhale, pull your opposite leg's heel to your bottom. Take hold of your foot with one hand and hold, drawing your navel into your spine and tucking your bottom under (posterior pelvic tilt)—do this by drawing your pubic bone up toward your sternum.

- If you find that your balance is challenged, place one hand on a chair for support.
- If you find that it is uncomfortable resting on your knee, place a cushion under your the knee or move your front leg farther forward so that you change the angle of your back leg, resting more on the top of the knee.
- Remain in this pose for up to three minutes. Try to maintain a smooth, lengthened breath.

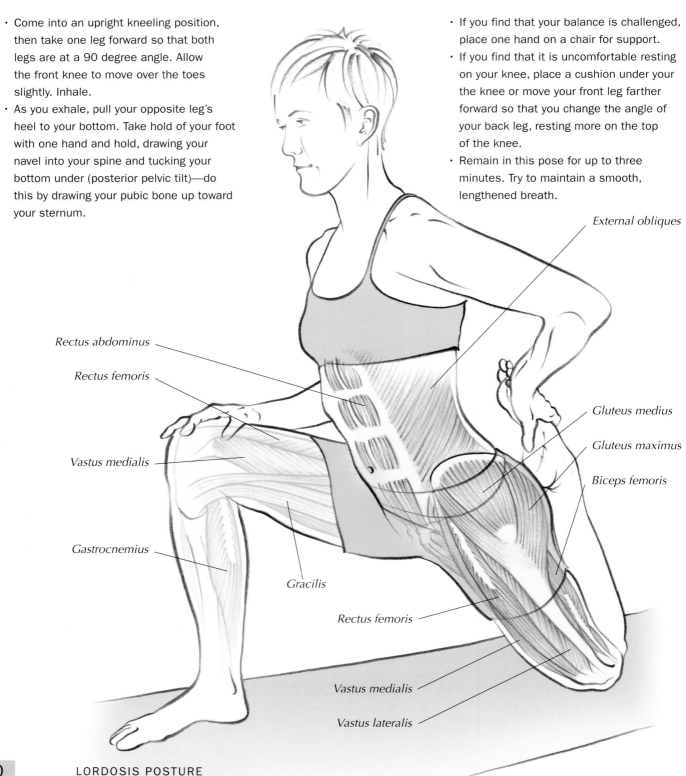

External obliques

Rectus abdominus

Rectus femoris

Vastus medialis

Gastrocnemius

Gracilis

Rectus femoris

Vastus medialis

Vastus lateralis

Gluteus medius

Gluteus maximus

Biceps femoris

LORDOSIS POSTURE

Modification

- Place one foot up against a wall. The closer your knee is to the wall, the stronger the stretch will be, so approach cautiously. Try to maintain a posterior pelvic tilt.

Benefits

- Improves flexibility in the front thighs. If the thigh muscles are shortened, especially the rectus femoris, it will affect the pull on the pelvis, creating imbalance. This stretch can also improve back complaints associated with an increased lumbar curve.

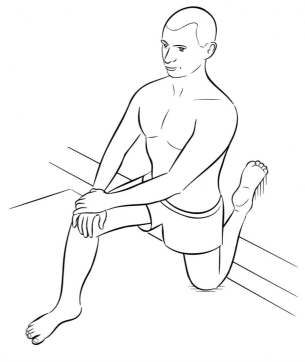

ANALYSIS OF MOVEMENT	JOINTS	JOINT MOVEMENT	MUSCLES ACTIVE	MUSCLES STRETCHED
Joint 1	Pelvis	Posterior pelvic tilt	Rectus abdominus, external and internal obliques, gluteus maximus, biceps femoris, semitendinosus, semimembranosus	Psoas major, possibly psoas minor
Joint 2	Hip	FL: flexion BL: extension	FL: rectus femoris, gluteus medius (anterior fibers), gluteus minimus, tensor fasciae latae, sartorius, psoas major, iliacus BL: biceps femoris, semitendinosus, semimembranosus, gluteus maximus, gluteus medius (posterior fibers), adductor magnus	FL: active for stabilization BL: psoas major, iliacus
Joint 3	Knee	Flexion	FL: biceps femoris, semitendinosus, semimembranosus, gracilis, sartorius, gastrocnemius, popliteus (isometrically), vastus and lateralis, rectus femoris BL: biceps femoris, semitendinosus, semimembranosus, gracilis	FL: working isometrically to stabilize BL: vastus medialis, lateralis, and intermedius, rectus femoris
Joint 4	Ankle	FL: dorsiflexion BL: plantarflexion	FL: tibialis anterior, extensor digitorum longus, extensor hallucis longus BL: the muscles for planterflexion should be passive due to the foot being held	BL: possibly tibialis anterior, extensor digitorum longus, extensor hallucis longus

(FL= front leg; BL = back leg)

KNEELING HIP FLEXOR STRETCH

Benefits

- This can help improve postural imbalances within pelvis alignment. It can also improve lower back pain when associated with increased lumbar curve.

- Come into an upright kneeling position, then step your right foot forward. Have your right leg at a right angle, with the knee directly over the ankle and the ankle vertical to the floor. The outer edge of your right knee should be in the same line as your outer right buttock.
- Your left knee should be placed directly under your left hip.
- Bring your attention to the pubic bone: draw it up toward your rib cage and simultaneously draw your tailbone down and under. This will assist the squeezing action of the left gluteus maximus muscle.
- Keep the upper torso lifted and lift the clavicles (collar bones).
- Remain in this pose for between two to three minutes, maintaining a smooth, even, diaphragmatic breath.

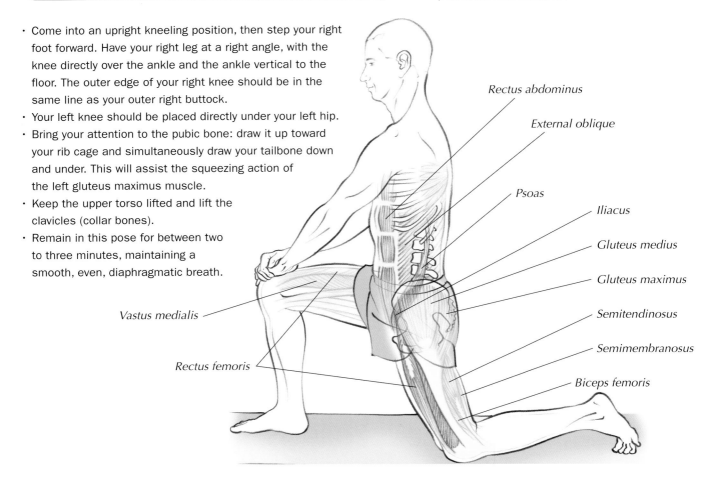

Rectus abdominus

External oblique

Psoas

Iliacus

Gluteus medius

Gluteus maximus

Semitendinosus

Semimembranosus

Biceps femoris

Vastus medialis

Rectus femoris

ANALYSIS OF MOVEMENT	JOINTS	JOINT MOVEMENT	MUSCLES ACTIVE	MUSCLES STRETCHED
Joint 1	Pelvis	Posterior pelvic tilt	Rectus abdominus, external and internal obliques, biceps femoris, gluteus maximus, gluteus medius (posterior fibers), semitendinosus, semimembranosus	
Joint 2	Hip	FL: flexion BL: extension	FL: rectus femoris, gluteus medius (anterior fibers), gluteus minimus, tensor fasciae latae, sartorius, psoas major, iliacus BL: biceps femoris, semitendinosus, semimembranosus, gluteus maximus, gluteus medius (posterior fibers), adductor magnus (posterior fibers)	FL: active for stabilization BL: psoas major, iliacus, rectus femoris

(FL= front leg; BL = back leg)

WARRIOR 1: VIRABHADRASANA (VARIATION 1)

- Take a wide stance with your feet parallel and turn your right foot out 90 degrees. Lift your left heel from the floor, taking it out so that your back foot also turns 90 degrees; your hips will naturally want to turn toward your right foot.
- If you find that your balance is challenged when starting this posture, use a chair to hold onto. Move your back foot toward the outer edge of your mat as if your feet were on train tracks, hip-width apart.
- Keeping your back leg straight, bend your front knee to a right angle. Do not allow the knee to go over the ankle.
- Inhale and roll your left inner thigh back, bringing your left hip forward.
- Exhale and press your right heel down and forward into the mat, as if pushing it away. Keep your right outer knee in line with your outer right hip.
- Inhale and press your back heel away from you and the back of the knee upward, straightening your leg.
- Exhale and, as in the previous stretch, draw up your pubic bone, activating the deep abdominal muscles while simultaneously dropping your tailbone down and under.

- Keep your torso facing the front. Inhale, roll your shoulders back, and take your arms back and interlace your fingers, straightening your arms and lifting them upward.
- Keep a steady breath and a connection with your feet.
- Remain in this pose for between two to three minutes, breathing diaphragmatically.

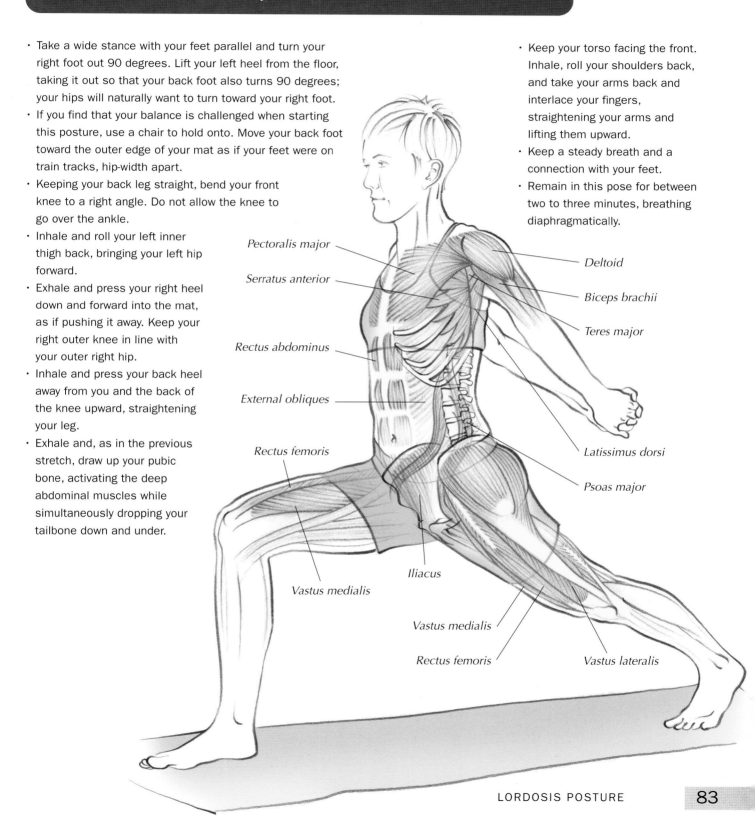

Pectoralis major

Serratus anterior

Rectus abdominus

External obliques

Rectus femoris

Vastus medialis

Iliacus

Vastus medialis

Rectus femoris

Deltoid

Biceps brachii

Teres major

Latissimus dorsi

Psoas major

Vastus lateralis

WARRIOR 1: VIRABHADRASANA (VARIATION 1)

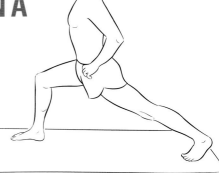

Benefits

· This classical asana has been changed to suit the postural imbalances of an excessive lumbar curve. It is effective in realigning a pelvic imbalance. It also aids digestion and strengthens the abdominals.

Modification

· Place your hands on your hips—this will help if your balance needs to be improved.

ANALYSIS OF MOVEMENT	JOINTS	JOINT MOVEMENT	MUSCLES ACTIVE	MUSCLES STRETCHED
Joint 1	Scapula	Downward rotation, adduction	Trapezius (middle fibers), rhomboid major and minor, levator scapula	Trapezius (upper and lower fibers), serratus anterior, pectoralis minor
Joint 2	Shoulder	Extension	Infraspinatus, teres minor, posterior deltoid, latissimus dorsi, teres major, pectoralis major (lower fibers)	Pectoralis major, anterior deltoid, biceps brachii, coracobracialis
Joint 3	Elbow	Extension, slight pronation	Triceps brachii, anconeus, pronator teres, pronator quadratus	
Joint 4	Spine	Extension	Spinalis, longissimus, ilicostalis, multifidi, rotatores, semispinalis capitis, intertransversarii, interspinalis, rectus abdominus, external and internal obliques	
Joint 5	Hip	FL: flexion BL: extension	FL: rectus femoris, gluteus medius (anterior fibers), gluteus minimus, tensor fasciae latae, sartorius, psoas major, iliacus BL: biceps femoris, semitendinosus, semimembranosus, gluteus maximus, gluteus medius (posterior fibers), adductor magnus (posterior fibers)	FL: active for stabilization BL: psoas major, iliacus, rectus femoris
Joint 6	Knee	FL: flexion BL: extension	FL: biceps femoris, semitendinosus, semimembranosus, gracilis, sartorius, gastrocnemius, popliteus (isometrically), vastus medialis and lateralis, rectus femoris BL: vastus medialis, lateralis and intermedius, rectus femoris	FL: active for stabilization BL: possibly rectus femoris
Joint 7	Ankle	Dorsiflexion	Tibialis anterior, extensor digitorum longus, extensor hallucis longus	BL: possibly gastrocnemius, soleus

(FL = front leg; BL = back leg)

HERO POSE: VIRASANA (VARIATION)

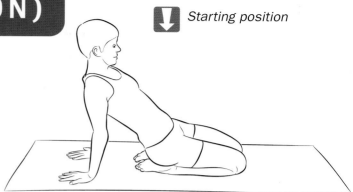

↓ *Starting position*

- Come to kneeling, bringing your inner knees together.
- Slowly lean back, taking your hands to the floor with your fingertips pointing away from your buttocks. At this point you may feel your lower back arch away from the floor—as in the previous asanas, draw your pubic bone toward your lower rib cage, simultaneously squeezing your buttocks and dropping your tailbone down and under, toward your knees.
- Stay in this pose for several breaths, then lift your buttocks away from your feet and push through your hands, lifting the chest and sternum at the same time. Roll the fronts of your shoulders back and to the floor.
- Allow your head to tip backward and place your tongue on the roof of your mouth to help support your neck.

- Maintain a steady, slow, even, diaphragmatic breath, remaining in the pose for up to three minutes.
- When coming out of the pose, lift your head slowly and make sure to keep your tongue on the roof of your mouth.

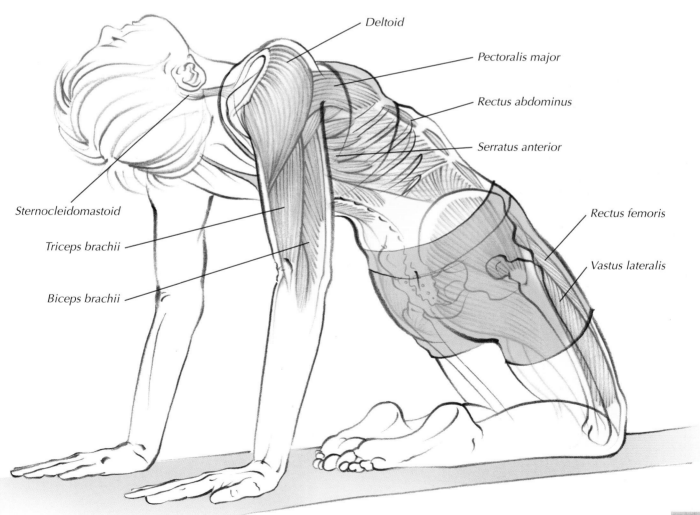

Deltoid

Pectoralis major

Rectus abdominus

Serratus anterior

Sternocleidomastoid

Triceps brachii

Biceps brachii

Rectus femoris

Vastus lateralis

HERO POSE: VIRASANA (VARIATION)

Benefits

· Increases flexibility in the chest and anterior shoulders and helps improve respiratory function. It can also improve digestion by increasing motility of internal organs.

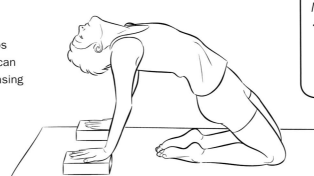

Modification

· Place your hands on blocks behind your hips; this will reduce the opening in the chest.

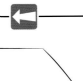

ANALYSIS OF MOVEMENT	JOINTS	JOINT MOVEMENT	MUSCLES ACTIVE	MUSCLES STRETCHED
Joint 1	Neck	Passive extension		Sternocleidomastoid, anterior scalene, longus capitus, longus coli
Joint 2	Scapula	Downward rotation, adduction	Trapezius (middle fibers), rhomboid major and minor, levator scapula	Trapezius (upper and lower fibers), serratus anterior, pectoralis minor
Joint 3	Shoulder	Extension, adduction, external rotation	Posterior deltoid, infraspinatus, teres minor, latissimus dorsi, teres major, pecotoralis major, triceps brachii (long head), coracobrachialis	Pectoralis major, anterior deltoid, biceps brachii, coracobracialis, serratus anterior, latissimus dorsi, teres major, subscapularis
Joint 4	Elbow	Extension, supination	Triceps brachii, anconeus, biceps brachii, supinator	Brachialis, brachioradialis, flexor carpi radialis, palmaris longus
Joint 5	Wrist	Passive extension		Flexor carpi radialis and ulnaris, palmaris longus, flexor digitorum superficialis and profundus
Joint 6	Spine	Extension	Spinalis, longissimus, ilicostalis, multifidi, rotatores, semispinalis capitis, intertransversarii, interspinalis, quadratus lumborum	Possibly rectus abdominus
Joint 7	Hip	Extension	Gluteus maximus, gluteus medius (posterior fibers), adductor magnus (posterior fibers)	Psoas major and minor, possibly iliacus, rectus femoris
Joint 8	Knee	Passive flexion		Rectus femoris, vastus lateralis, intermedius and medialis
Joint 9	Ankle	Passive plantarflexion		Possibly tibialis anterior, extensor digitorum longus, extensor hallucis longus

CHILD'S POSE: BALASANA VARIATION

Benefits
- Releases tension in the hips and lower back while the arms, neck, and head rest. It is used frequently in yoga practice as a restful pose. It is also said to relieve abdominal bloating and alleviate gas.

- Remaining in the kneeling position from the previous asana, nestle your buttocks onto your heels. Keep that connection and then walk your hands forward until your arms are straight and your elbows are off the floor.
- With your arms outstretched, walk your left hand just to the outside of the mat, then place your right hand over the top of your left hand, interlacing your fingers.
- Reach both arms forward as you keep your right buttock nestled to your right heel, allowing your forehead to rest on the floor. Breathe into your abdomen.
- Remain in the pose for up to three minutes on each side.

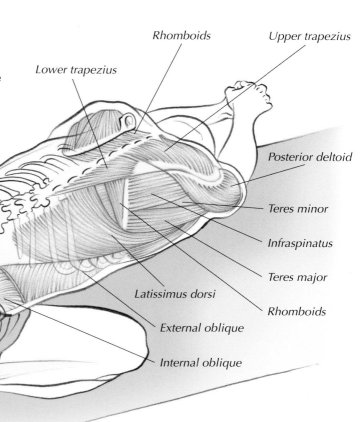

Lower trapezius
Rhomboids
Upper trapezius
Posterior deltoid
Teres minor
Infraspinatus
Teres major
Latissimus dorsi
Rhomboids
External oblique
Internal oblique
Gluteus medius
Gluteus maximus

ANALYSIS OF MOVEMENT	JOINTS	JOINT MOVEMENT	MUSCLES ACTIVE	MUSCLES STRETCHED
Joint 1	Scapula	Upward rotation, abduction	Trapezius (upper and lower fibers), serratus anterior, pectoralis minor	Trapezius (middle fibers), rhomboid minor and major
Joint 2	Shoulder	Flexion, internal rotation, adduction	Anterior deltoid, pectoralis major, biceps brachii, coracobrachialis, teres major, subscapularis, infraspinatus, teres minor, triceps brachii (long head)	Latissimus dorsi, teres minor, infraspinatus, posterior deltoid
Joint 3	Spine	Passive flexion, active rotation to the lower arm side	Multifidi, rotatores, external and internal obliques	
Joint 4	Hip	Deep passive flexion		Gluteus maximus, gluteus medius (posterior fibers)

PLANK

Modification
- Keep your knees on the floor, but still maintain the main teaching points.

- Lie on your front and place your elbows directly under your shoulders, with your wrists in line with your elbows. Lift your chest from the floor, draw your shoulder blades down, away from your ears, and maintain that connection throughout.
- Tuck your toes under.
- On your exhalation, push up with your forearms and knees, making the spine parallel to the floor so that only your forearms and toes are on the floor.
- Press your forearms down and forward into the mat. Lift your armpits and keep your shoulder blades moving down toward the sacrum. Press your heels back and keep your neck long and your chin slightly retracted, with the crown of your head reaching forward.

- Make sure that your navel is tightly drawn in and your tailbone is drawn to your heels, creating a slight posterior pelvic tilt.
- Keep a constant slow breath: this will help maintain energetic alignment and strength.
- Build up gradually until you can hold the pose for four minutes. Be aware of your alignment; if you feel yourself start to weaken, come out of the pose. Do not hold the pose with poor alignment, as this can put excessive strain on the lower back.

Benefits
- Improves upper body and abdominal strength.

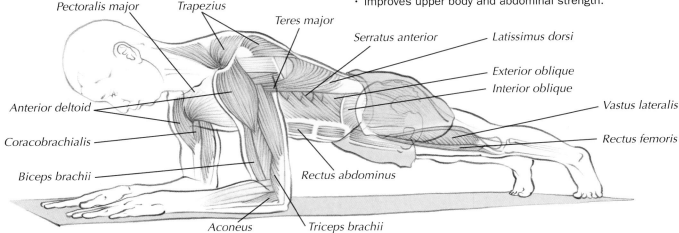

Pectoralis major — Trapezius — Teres major — Serratus anterior — Latissimus dorsi — Exterior oblique — Interior oblique — Vastus lateralis — Anterior deltoid — Coracobrachialis — Rectus femoris — Biceps brachii — Rectus abdominus — Aconeus — Triceps brachii

ANALYSIS OF MOVEMENT	JOINTS	JOINT MOVEMENT	MUSCLES ACTIVE
Joint 1	Neck	Extension	Trapezius (upper fibers), levator scapula, splenius capitis, splenius cervicis, rectus capitis posterior major and minor, oblique capitis superior, semispinalis capitis
Joint 2	Scapula	Upward rotation, abduction	Trapezius (upper and lower fibers), serratus anterior, pectoralis minor
Joint 3	Shoulder	Flexion, internal rotation, horizontal adduction	Anterior deltoid, pectoralis major, biceps brachii, coracobrachialis, teres major, subscapularis, latissimus dorsi
Joint 4	Elbow	Passive flexion moving to extension	Triceps brachii, aconeus
Joint 5	Spine	Active neutral	Spinalis, longissimus, ilicostalis, multifidi, rotatores, semispinalis capitis, intertransversarii, interspinalis, quadratus lumborum, rectus abdominus, external and internal obliques, transverse abdominus
Joint 6	Hip	Active neutral	Biceps femoris, semitendinosus, semimembranosus, pectineus, adductor brevis, longus, and magnus

LEG DROPS

- Lie on your back with your arms by your sides, palms down. Bend your knees and place your feet flat on the floor.
- Draw both knees directly over your hips.
- Exhale and draw your navel in toward your spine, pressing your lumbar spine to the floor and your tailbone toward the ceiling.
- With your knees bent and your lower back pressing to the floor, exhale and lower your feet with control to the floor. Inhale as you pause at the bottom, hovering your feet just above the floor, then exhale and bring them back to the starting position.
- Repeat this movement with a steady breath 15 to 20 times.
- Make sure that you keep your lower back in contact with the floor at all times.

Benefits
- Increases strength in the abdominal region. Also helps improve postural imbalance within the pelvic region in association with an increased lumbar curve.

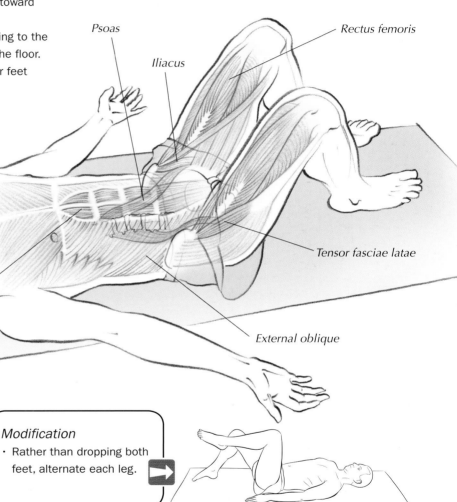

Psoas

Rectus femoris

Iliacus

Tensor fasciae latae

Rectus abdominus

External oblique

Starting position

Modification
- Rather than dropping both feet, alternate each leg.

ANALYSIS OF MOVEMENT	JOINTS	JOINT MOVEMENT	MUSCLES ACTIVE
Joint 1	Lumbar spine	Flexion	Rectus abdominus, external and internal obliques
Joint 2	Hip	Flexion, adduction	Rectus femoris, gluteus medius (anterior fibers), gluteus minimus, adductor magnus, adductor longus, pectineus, tensor fasciae latae, sartorius, psoas major, iliacus, gracilis
Joint 3	Knee	Passive flexion to extension	Rectus femoris, vastus lateralis, medialis, and intermedius

LEG ROLLS

- Lie on your back with your arms at shoulder height, palms up.
- Bring your knees above your hips, push your lower back into the floor, and straighten your legs perpendicular to the floor. Keep your legs straight and stiff and your inner thighs tight together, with your feet flexed.
- As you exhale, lower your legs to the right until the toes of your right foot are almost touching your right hand. Both legs should go down together, with the knees kept tight.
- When your legs are near your outstretched arm, move the left side of your rib cage to the left and press your left shoulder and arm to the floor, resisting the urge to lift your left side from the floor.
- Stay in this position with your legs together and completely straight for up to two minutes, then slowly return to the center and repeat on the opposite side. Pull your navel to your spine throughout. Repeat the pose on each side between one and three times.

Benefits
- Increases strength in abdominal region. It helps improve postural imbalance within the pelvic region in association with an increased lumbar curve. It also improves rotational mobility in the spine.

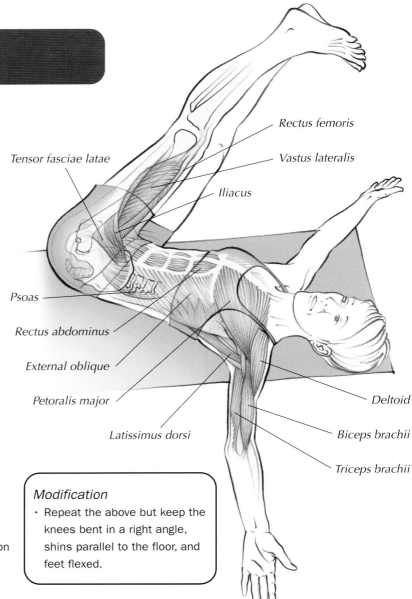

Tensor fasciae latae

Rectus femoris

Vastus lateralis

Iliacus

Psoas

Rectus abdominus

External oblique

Petoralis major

Latissimus dorsi

Deltoid

Biceps brachii

Triceps brachii

Modification
- Repeat the above but keep the knees bent in a right angle, shins parallel to the floor, and feet flexed.

ANALYSIS OF MOVEMENT	JOINTS	JOINT MOVEMENT	MUSCLES ACTIVE
Joint 1	Scapula	Downward rotation, adduction	Rhomboid major and minor, levator scapula
Joint 2	Shoulder	Horizontal abduction, external rotation, extension	Deltoid (posterior fibers), latissimus dorsi, teres major, subscapularis, pectoralis major, teres minor, infraspinatus, triceps brachii (long head), supraspinatus
Joint 3	Spine	Flexion, rotation	Rectus abdominus, transversus abdominus, external and internal obliques, mutifidi, rotatores
Joint 4	Hip	Flexion, adduction	Rectus femoris, gluteus medius (anterior fibers), gluteus minimus, adductor magnus, longus and brevis, pectineus, tensor fasciae latae, sartorius, psoas major, iliacus, gracilis
Joint 5	Knee	Extension	Rectus femoris, vastus lateralis, medialis, and intermedius

CORPSE POSE: SAVASANA

"Sava" means corpse; this is a deep relaxation pose where the body is motionless, appearing like a corpse. We spend most of our daily lives moving, rarely enjoying stillness; practicing this pose provides the time to experience deep stillness and inner calm. Concentrate your mind on the subtle movements of your breath and the rise and fall of the abdomen. On each exhalation, have a sense of letting go of tension, allowing the body to surrender to gravity. Try not to get caught in unnecessary thoughts. Just allow the body to be.

- Start on your back with your heels toward the sitting bones, then gently straighten one leg at a time. Stretch your legs away from you, draw the pubic bone toward you for a second, lengthening the lower back, then relax.
- Have your legs a little wider than hip-width apart. Straighten your arms away from your body, palms up, and relax your shoulders away from your ears. Lengthen your head away from your shoulders.
- Soften the skin of your face and let your jaw part slightly.

- Rest here for between five and ten minutes.
- When you have finished, roll onto your right side, rest here for a few moments, and open your eyes, then gently bring yourself into a sitting position, becoming aware of your surroundings.
- If you find tension gathering in your neck, place a small blanket underneath your neck to help keep it lengthened. You may also place a blanket underneath your knees to take any stress out of your lower back. An eyemask can be used on the eyes, as this is effective in calming the nervous system.

Benefits

- "Lying upon one's back on the ground at full length like a corpse removes fatigue caused by the other asana and induces calmness of mind" (S. Muktibodhananda, *Hatha Yoga Pradipika*). This posture gives the body time to relax and enjoy stillness and has a calming effect on the nervous system.

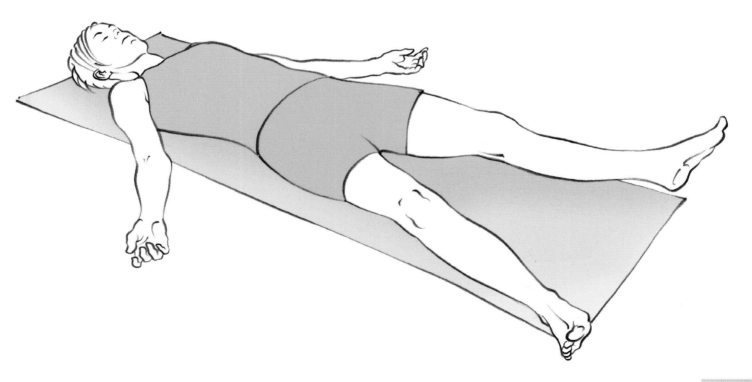

The tendency to have an excessive curve in the lumbar spine with a lordotic posture can coincide with weakness in the lower abdominal area. The following practice can help awaken a connection with the transversus abdominis and pelvic floor. Another benefit of lengthening your exhalation is a spontaneous deepening of the inhalation; as your exhalation lengthens, there is a dramatic effect on the parasympathetic nervous system, taking you into a more restful and calm state.

Three-part exhalation

Assume a position that is comfortable for you. This practice can be done seated (see page 38 for variations) or kneeling or lying on your back. For the purpose of these instructions we will use an easy crossed-leg position. Place a blanket or a block underneath your buttocks and slide forward, raising the sitting bones just off the blanket while leaving the flesh of your buttocks still on the blanket. Lengthen your spine—imagine the crown of your head floating upward and your chin slightly dropping down and back toward the throat.

Stretch your arms out straight and rest the backs of your hands on your knees. Join the tips of your index fingers with the tips of your thumbs and straighten the remaining three fingers—this is known as jnana mudra, the seal of knowledge. The index finger represents the individual soul and the thumb represents the universal soul; the union of the two symbolizes knowledge.

Relax your neck, shoulders and facial muscles. Bring your awareness to your breath: the tempo, quality, and direction. Do not change this once observed, just spend time connecting with every aspect, allowing the breath to be. Stay with this for a few minutes, bringing the mind and body together in union. Start to bring your attention to your exhalation. Observe the exhalation length, then gradually start to lengthen the exhalation into three equal parts: visualize the breath descending from throat to heart and pause; from heart to navel and pause; and from navel to pubic bone and pause. During the last phase, draw the belly button into the spine and lift your pelvic floor.

As you start the inhalation, release the pelvic floor. Let the inhalation be a comfortable length—don't force it. The pauses between the sections of breath should be more like a moment of hesitation rather than a holding of your breath. Continue with this rhythm for 10 to 15 rounds. Throughout the practice, focus on remaining upright in the spine, shoulders, and neck and always keep your jaw relaxed. It also helps if you keep your eyes closed, internalizing your awareness.

MEDITATION PRACTICE: GROUNDING MEDITATION

A great part of our daily lives is spent thinking about what has to be done and what hasn't been done. Sometimes this can get overwhelming, and we can experience a sense of wanting everything to slow down or stop so that we can breathe again. The grounding meditation is an effective way of helping the mind and body to calm down, creating space in between the incessant chatter of the mind.

As with the other mediations in this book, we suggest that you speak slowly and clearly into a recorder. If this doesn't suit you, read the meditation a few times so that you get the journey in your mind. Then create your own meditation in your own words.

This meditation can also be done sitting on a chair, with your feet placed firmly on the floor.

The practice

Settle yourself into a sitting pose and take a few moments to calm your mind and body. Scan your body from head to toe, become aware of any areas that may feel uncomfortable, and move them. Move your awareness now to your breath: become aware of the quality and the length, then breathe into your muscles, bones, and organs until you feel calm.

Start to become aware of the areas of your body that connect with the floor. Spend a few moments feeling every area of this connection and start to imagine roots growing out of these connection points extending slowly through the floor and into the earth. Watch them move deeper and deeper until they hit the magnetic core. Allow your body to feel the effects of this. Let your body surrender to the pull of the roots. Feel all tension, stress, and negative emotions drain out of the body into the roots and away from you. Breathe evenly and softly. Now that your body has relaxed, imagine a ball of healing earth energy gathering at the bottom of your roots and starting to move up your roots toward your body. Take as long as you need to imagine the energy moving toward you. As it comes closer to your body, visualize it moving through your limbs, permeating every cell, muscle, and bone. As it reaches your abdomen, let it pause there for a moment.

As you rest here, focus on this energy and observe any physical, emotional, or mental effects this has on you. Immerse yourself in these feelings. When you are ready, visualize this ball of energy slowly expanding, enveloping you as if in a bubble. Feel its protection and know that you are in a safe environment. Pause here, embracing this feeling of safety and connection to the earth. You can stay in this space for as long as you need.

After a period of time, maintaining the sense of being surrounded by a grounding, protective bubble, start to take a few deep breaths, bringing your mind and body back to your surroundings. Swallow to become aware of taste, wiggle your toes and fingers, then slowly stretch your body in whichever way you feel you want to, gradually opening your eyes. When you are ready, move forward into your day knowing that you have roots feeding you healing energy.

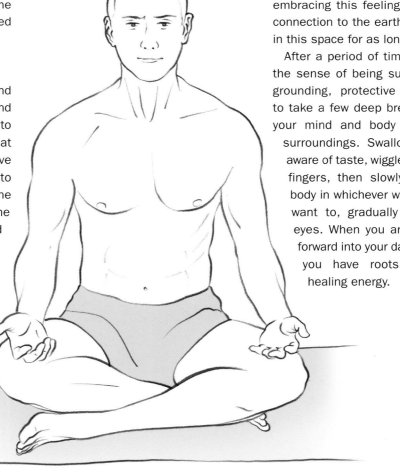

FLAT-BACK POSTURE

A flat-back posture is one where the lumbar spine reduces its curvature to less than 30 degrees and the L1 vertebra effectively moves farther away from the L5 vertebra.

In addition to the decrease in lumbar curvature, there is normally a concomitant posterior rotation of the pelvis and extension of the hip joints.

The thoracic spine will compensate above it to maintain the center of gravity by increasing its kyphosis, especially the top of the thoracic spine, causing the head to move forward. The knees can hyperextend or flex.

With a flat-back posture, there will be a tightening of the hamstrings and possibly also of the lower abdominals. There is also lengthening and weakening of the iliopsoas muscles.

Physical causes

A flat-back posture can be caused by a number of factors. These include:

- Sitting slumped for long periods with the lumbar spine flexed
- Sports in which one spends long periods of time in a flexed position such as:
    - Rowing
    - Cycling
    - Car racing
- Jobs that require long periods spent bending forward such as:
    - Car mechanic
    - Dentist
    - Delivery driver
    - Surgeon
- Weak deep abdominal wall
- Sacro-iliac joint dysfunction
- Wearing high-heeled shoes

Emotional causes

What is apparent with this particular postural type is the flat lumbar spine. This can be coupled with a strong, inflexible abdominal area. The result of this will affect the flow of emotions through the belly, an area of the body known to store emotions that haven't yet been dealt with. "When an emotion is blocked before it is fully

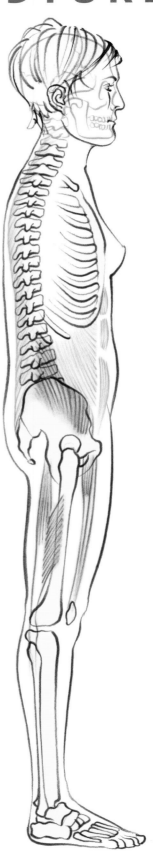

expressed, the energetic charge of the emotion and of the experience that gave birth to the emotion seems to become stressfully trapped within the part of the bodymind that corresponds to the blockage" (K. Dychtwald, *Bodymind*).

A further consideration is that the tension in the abdominal region can consequently disturb the function of the diaphragm, which can affect optimal breathing patterns. As discussed on pages 34 and 35, if the breath is uneven and erractic, the mind fluctuations will follow.

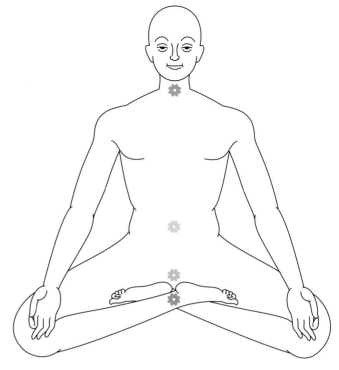

Forward head	Posterior pelvic tilt	Lower back tightness	Tight hamstrings
Encounter the world first with their head	Lessening of sexual energy and holding of sexual feelings	Extremely compulsive	Related to self-control
	Inability to stay grounded in emotional activity		Difficulty letting go
	Feelings are constricted or constrained		Fears of being abandoned
			Fears of loss of support

Chakra	Positive feelings cultivated	Location	Bija mantra
Root chakra/1st—muladhara	Grounding Inner strength Stability	Perineum, below the genitals and above the anus inside the coccyx; related to the pelvic plexus	Lam
Sacral chakra/ 2nd—svadhistahana	Self-love Worthy of love Acceptance of how perfect you are	Genital area, hypogastric plexus	Vam
Solar plexus chakra/ 3rd—manipura	Self-confidence Courage Fearless of life's challenges	The part of the vertebral column that relates to the navel; solar plexus	Ram
Throat chakra/5th—vishuddha	Truthful speech Honesty to oneself Freedom of self-expression	The neck region; the cervical part of the spinal column, related to the throat; carotid plexus	Ham

EXPANDED LEG FORWARD BEND: PRASARITA PADOTTANASANA

- Spread your legs 4–5 ft. (1–1.5 m) apart and have your feet parallel with each other and each foot pointing forward. Settle your weight evenly between the balls and heels of your feet.
- Press your heels down into the mat and slightly out. Without moving them, simultaneously press the big toe joints down and in.
- Roll your upper inner thighs back, feeling your buttocks spread as you do this.
- As you exhale, pivot forward at your hips, bending your knees just enough to maintain an anterior tilt in your pelvis: this is achieved by lifting the sitting bones upward.

Starting position

Benefits
- Increases flexibility in the hips and can improve mobility in the lumbar spine and pelvis.

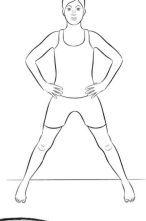

- As the spine comes parallel to the floor, place your hands on the floor directly under your shoulders. Extend forward with the crown of your head, so that your gaze is between your hands. Stay here for several breaths.
- If you feel your hamstrings start to ease and wish to take if farther, you can start to straighten your legs. Initiate this movement by raising the sitting bones rather than by pressing back your knees.
- Remain in this pose for between two and three minutes, breathing diaphragmatically.
- To come out of this pose, bend your knees deeply and gently roll up on an inhalation.

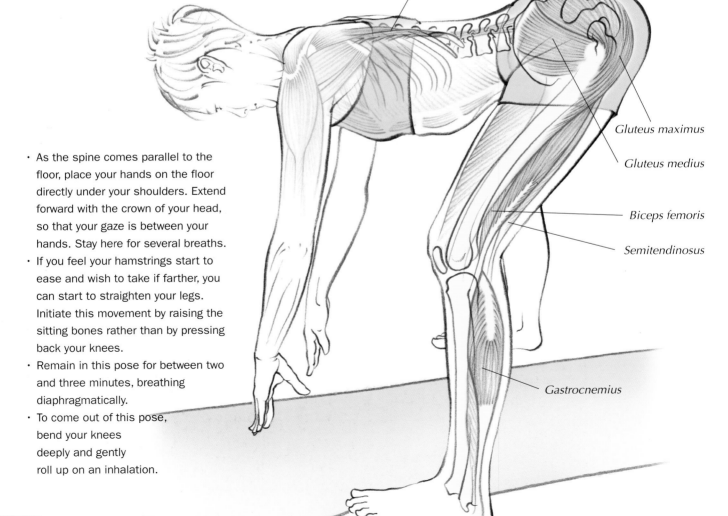

Spinalis, longissimus, ilicostalis

Gluteus maximus

Gluteus medius

Biceps femoris

Semitendinosus

Gastrocnemius

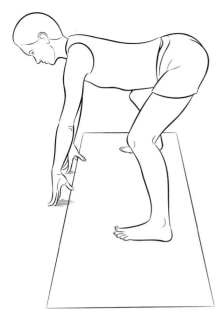

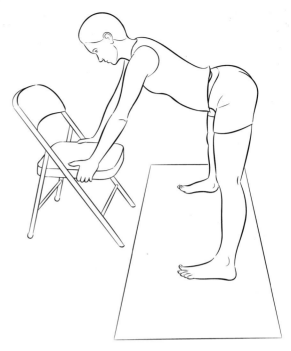

Modification 1
· Follow the same instructions, but bend your knees a little more and touch no more than your fingertips to the floor.

Modification 2
· Place a chair in front of you and follow the same teaching points but place your hands on the chair.

ANALYSIS OF MOVEMENT	JOINTS	JOINT MOVEMENT	MUSCLES ACTIVE	MUSCLES STRETCHED
Joint 1	Spine	Concentric extension	Spinalis, longissimus, ilicostalis, multifidi, rotatores, semispinalis capitis, intertransversarii, interspinalis, quadratus lumborum	
Joint 2	Hip	Flexion, abduction	Rectus femoris, tensor fasciae latae, sartorius, psoas major iliacus, gluteus minimus, gluteus medius (anterior fibers), gluteus maximus	Gluteus maximus (lower fibers), gluteus medius (posterior fibers), adductor magnus, minimus, longus and brevis, gracilis, biceps femoris, semitendinosus, semimembranosus
Joint 3	Knee	Extension	Vastus lateralis, medialis and intermedius, rectus femoris	Possibly gastrocnemius
Joint 4	Ankle	Inversion	Tibialis anterior and posterior, flexor digitorum longus, flexor hallucis longus, extensor hallucis longus	Peroneus longus and brevis, extensor digitorum longus

INTENSE SIDE STRETCH: PARSVOTTANASANA (VARIATION)

- Step your feet apart one-leg's distance, then turn your right foot 90 degrees and your left foot about 45 degrees—do this by lifting your heel and shifting it outward.
- Your hips will naturally want to turn to the right; allow this to happen until both hips are facing toward your right foot. Your right hip will move back as your left hip moves forward to come into the same plane (see starting position illustration).
- Press your front heel down and inward with your big toe down and outward, without moving the foot. Keep the heel on your back foot down and out, with the big toe joint down and in, which in turn will roll your left hip forward in line with your right.

Starting position ➡

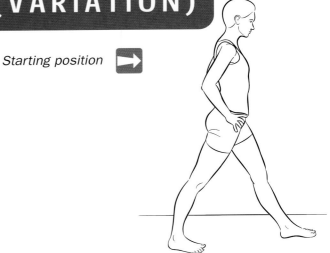

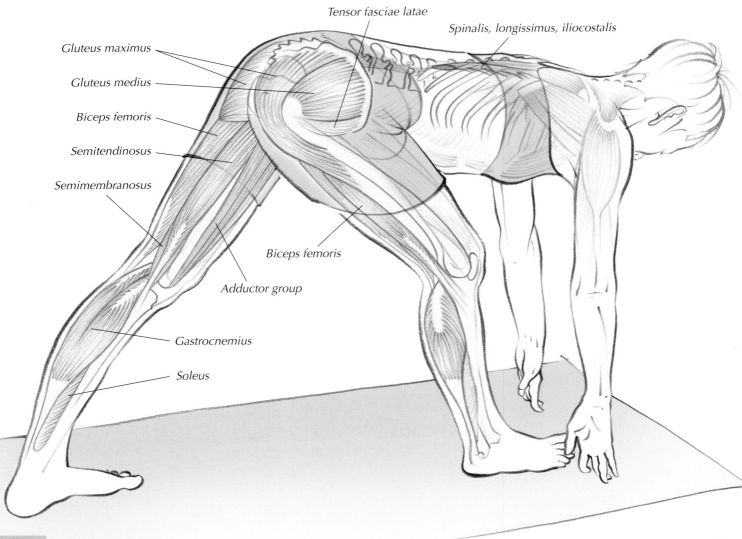

Tensor fasciae latae

Spinalis, longissimus, iliocostalis

Gluteus maximus

Gluteus medius

Biceps femoris

Semitendinosus

Semimembranosus

Biceps femoris

Adductor group

Gastrocnemius

Soleus

- Bend your right knee about 45 degrees, lift your sitting bones, and hinge forward at the hips, taking your hands down onto the floor. Keep your feet active and maintain a lumbar curve. Keep the heels pressing away from each other.
- You should be able to take one hand back to your sacrum to feel that both hips are in line, so much so that you could balance a glass of water there.
- The back of the neck should stay long—extend forward with the crown of your head, retracting your chin slightly to the throat. Hold this pose for up to two minutes, maintaining a neutral spine throughout. If you feel your hamstrings beginning to release, progress to straightening your front leg and hold the pose for a further minute, maintaining the action in the feet.

Benefits
- Increases flexibility in the hamstrings, improving lumbar mobility, and improves balance and coordination.

Modification
- Use blocks, still keeping a strong connection, with your feet driving apart.

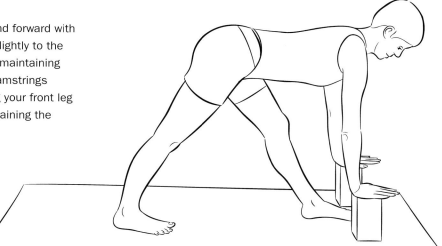

ANALYSIS OF MOVEMENT	JOINTS	JOINT MOVEMENT	MUSCLES ACTIVE	MUSCLES STRETCHED
Joint 1	Spine	Concentric extension	Spinalis, longissimus, ilicostalis, multifidi, rotatores, semispinalis capitis, intertransversarii, interspinalis, quadratus lumborum	
Joint 2	Hip	Flexion; back leg also has medial rotation	Rectus femoris, gluteus medius (anterior fibers), gluteus minimus, tensor fasciae latae, sartorius, psoas major, iliacus; back leg would also have activity of semitendinosus, semimembranosus, adductor magnus, longus, and brevis, gracilis, pectineus, tensor fasciae latae	Gluteus maximus (lower fibers), gluteus medius (posterior fibers), biceps femoris, semitendinosus, semimembranosus
Joint 3	Knee	Extension	Rectus femoris, vastus lateralis, medialis, and intermedius	Gastrocnemius, plantaris
Joint 4	Ankle	Dorsiflexion	Tibialis anterior, extensor digitorum longus, extensor hallucis longus	Gastrocnemius, soleus

EXTENDED STRAIGHT LEG STRETCH: UTTHITA HASTA PADANGUSTHASANA (VARIATION)

- Standing with your feet together, ground through your feet by pressing evenly through the toes and heels of both feet.
- Place your hands on your hips, gaze at a point in front of you, and focus on that point. Shift your weight to the left foot, inhale, and bring your right knee to hip height. Hold here for a few breaths, then, on an exhalation, gradually straighten your leg to hip height, pointing the toe forward.
- Maintain an erect spine with your chest lifted and hips in line.
- Focus on a smooth, even, diaphragmatic breath. Gradually build up to holding the pose for one to two minutes.

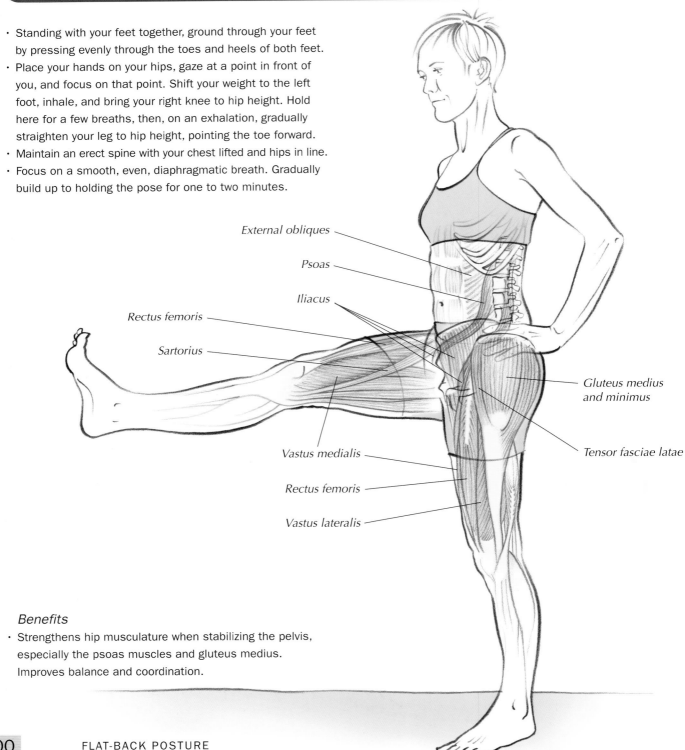

External obliques

Psoas

Iliacus

Rectus femoris

Sartorius

Gluteus medius and minimus

Tensor fasciae latae

Vastus medialis

Rectus femoris

Vastus lateralis

Benefits
- Strengthens hip musculature when stabilizing the pelvis, especially the psoas muscles and gluteus medius. Improves balance and coordination.

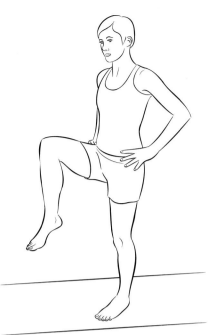

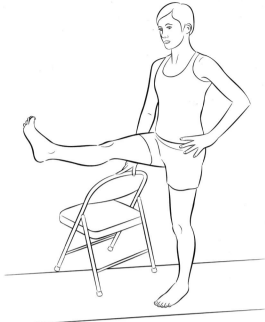

Modification 1
· Until you build up strength and balance, keep the leg bent, gradually building the flexibility and strength of the abdominals and hip flexors to straighten the leg.

Modification 2
· Use a chair for balance until you build up enough strength to try the pose unassisted.

ANALYSIS OF MOVEMENT	JOINTS	JOINT MOVEMENT	MUSCLES ACTIVE	MUSCLES STRETCHED
Joint 1	Spine	Extension	Spinalis, longissimus, ilicostalis, multifidi, rotatores, semispinalis capitis, intertransversarii, interspinalis, quadratus lumborum, external and internal obliques	
Joint 2	Hip	SL: abduction, external rotation LL: flexion	SL: gluteus maximus, gluteus medius, gluteus minimus, tensor fasciae latae, sartorius LL: rectus femoris, gluteus medius (anterior fibers), gluteus minimus, tensor fasciae latae, sartorius, psoas major, iliacus	LL: gluteus maximus, semitendinosus, semimembranosus, biceps femoris
Joint 3	Knee	Extension	Rectus femoris, vastus lateralis, vastus medialis, vastus intermedius	Gastrocnemius, soleus
Joint 4	Ankle	Dorsiflexion	Tibialis anterior, extensor digitorum longus, extensor hallucis longus	

(SL = standing leg; LL = lifted leg)

WARRIOR 1: VIRABHADRASANA (VARIATION 2)

- Take a wide stance, with your feet parallel. Turn your right foot out 90 degrees, then lift your left heel from the floor so that your foot turns 90 degrees; both hips will turn toward your right foot.
- If you find that your balance is challenged here, move the back foot toward the outer edge of your mat as if your feet were on train tracks, hip-width apart.
- Bend your front knee to a right angle. Do not allow the knee to go over the ankle. Come onto the toes of your back foot and bend the knee toward the floor.
- Press your right heel down and forward but also slightly inward, without actually moving the foot. This will naturally move your big toe base down and outward, which will keep your outer knee in line with your outer hip. Maintain pressure through your heel to the floor, as if you are on a scale and trying to increase the weight.
- Draw up your pubic bone, activating the deep abdominal muscles, while simultaneously dropping your tailbone down and under.
- Keep your torso to the front. Put your hands behind your back and interlace your fingers, press the heels of your hands together, and lift your arms.
- Gradually build up to holding the pose for three minutes. Maintain at all times a smooth, even, diaphragmatic breath.

Benefits

- This classical asana has been altered to suit the postural imbalances of an excessively flattened lumbar spine. The priority is to increase strength in the gluteus maximus. If the back leg were to straighten, this would increase the openness to the front of the hips even more, but this is not the primary objective. This asana can help aid digestion and strengthen the abdominals.

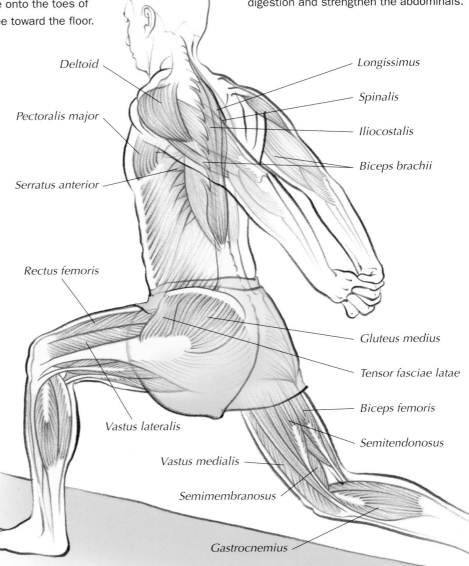

Deltoid

Pectoralis major

Serratus anterior

Rectus femoris

Vastus lateralis

Vastus medialis

Semimembranosus

Gastrocnemius

Longissimus

Spinalis

Iliocostalis

Biceps brachii

Gluteus medius

Tensor fasciae latae

Biceps femoris

Semitendonosus

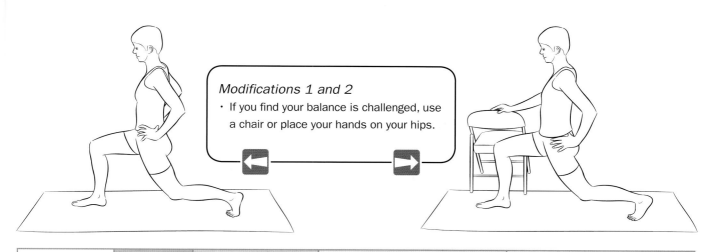

Modifications 1 and 2
· If you find your balance is challenged, use a chair or place your hands on your hips.

ANALYSIS OF MOVEMENT	JOINTS	JOINT MOVEMENT	MUSCLES ACTIVE	MUSCLES STRETCHED
Joint 1	Scapula	Downward rotation, adduction	Rhomboid major, rhomboid minor, levator scapula	Serratus anterior, pectoralis minor, trapezius (upper and lower fibers)
Joint 2	Shoulder	Extension	Infraspinatus, teres minor, posterior deltoid, latissimus dorsi, teres major, pectoralis major (lower fibers), trapezius, rhomboids	Pectoralis major, anterior deltoid, biceps brachii, coracobracialis, serratus anterior
Joint 3	Elbow	Extension, slight pronation	Triceps brachii, anconeus, pronator teres, pronator quadratus	
Joint 4	Spine	Extension	Spinalis, longissimus, ilicostalis, multifidi, rotatores, semispinalis capitis, intertransversarii, interspinalis, rectus abdominus, external and internal obliques, transverse abdominus	
Joint 5	Hip	FL: flexion BL: extension	FL: rectus femoris, gluteus medius (anterior fibers), gluteus minimus, tensor fasciae latae, sartorius, psoas major, iliacus BL: biceps femoris, semitendinosus, semimembranosus, gluteus maximus and medius (posterior fibers), adductor magnus (posterior fibers)	FL: active for stabilization only BL: psoas major, iliacus, rectus femoris
Joint 6	Knee	FL: flexion BL: extension	FL: biceps femoris, semitendinosus, semimembranosus, gracilis, sartorius, gastrocnemius, popliteus (isometrically), vastus medialis, vastus lateralis, rectus femoris BL: vastus medialis, vastus lateralis, rectus femoris, vastus intermedius	FL: active for stabilization only BL: possibly rectus femoris
Joint 7	Ankle	Dorsiflexion	Tibialis anterior, extensor digitorum longus, extensor hallucis longus	BL: possibly gastrocnemius, soleus

(FL = front leg; BL = back leg)

SUPINE FOOT TOE POSE: SUPTA PADANGUSTAHASANA

- Place a small rolled towel underneath your lumbar spine to create a curve. The towel (when compressed) should be the width and thickness of the fattest part of your hand.
- Extend your heels away from you and broaden across your upper back. Inhale and, as you exhale, draw your right knee toward your chest. Take hold of your big toe with the first two fingers of your right hand.

- Press your left hand onto the top of your left thigh, encouraging the grounding of your left thigh.
- On your next inhalation, straighten your right leg to the ceiling while still holding your big toe. Keep length in the back of your neck and relax your shoulders while keeping your hips in the same place.
- Remain in the pose for up to three minutes, all the while extending the left heel away and the right heel up.

Benefits
- By placing a towel under the lumber spine, it encourages an anterior tilt of the pelvis; this will create a more effective stretch on the hamstrings, improving the mobility of lumbar spine. The pose also increases flexibility in the hips.

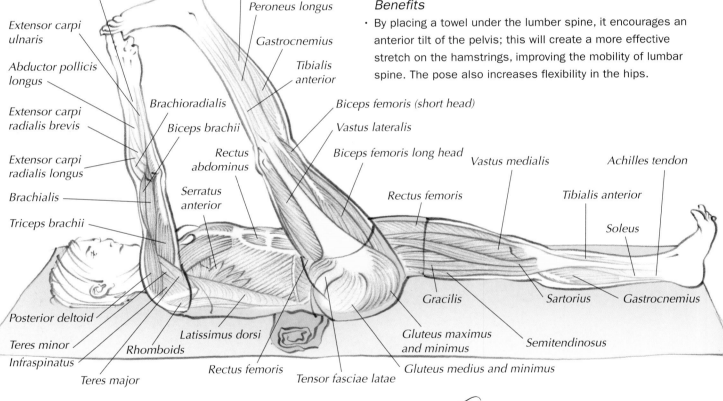

Extensor digitorum

Extensor carpi ulnaris

Abductor pollicis longus

Extensor carpi radialis brevis

Extensor carpi radialis longus

Brachialis

Triceps brachii

Posterior deltoid

Teres minor

Infraspinatus

Teres major

Brachioradialis

Biceps brachii

Rectus abdominus

Serratus anterior

Latissimus dorsi

Rhomboids

Rectus femoris

Tensor fasciae latae

Soleus

Peroneus longus

Gastrocnemius

Tibialis anterior

Biceps femoris (short head)

Vastus lateralis

Biceps femoris long head

Rectus femoris

Gracilis

Gluteus maximus and minimus

Gluteus medius and minimus

Vastus medialis

Achilles tendon

Tibialis anterior

Soleus

Sartorius

Gastrocnemius

Semitendinosus

Modification 1
- If you have difficulty holding the big toe, use a strap, looping it around the ball of the foot.

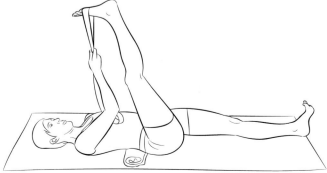

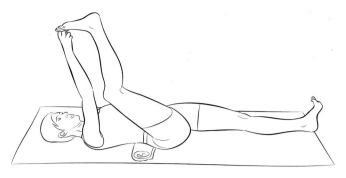

> **Modification 2**
> · Bend the knee slightly if you find the stretch too strong with the leg straight. →

ANALYSIS OF MOVEMENT	JOINTS	JOINT MOVEMENT	MUSCLES ACTIVE	MUSCLES STRETCHED
Joint 1	Scapula	TA: upward rotation, abduction BA: downward rotation, adduction	TA: trapezius (upper and lower fibers), serratus anterior, pectoralis minor BA: rhomboid major and minor, levator scapula	
Joint 2	Shoulder	TA: flexion BA: extension, adduction	TA: anterior deltoid, pectoralis major, biceps brachii, coracobrachialis, BA: infraspinatus, teres minor, posterior deltoid, anterior deltoid, pectoralis major (lower fibers), latissimus dorsi, teres major	
Joint 3	Elbow	TA: extension BA: extension, pronation	TA: triceps brachii, aconeus BA: triceps brachii, aconeus, pronator teres, pronator quadratus, brachioradialis	
Joint 4	Spine	Active neutral	Transverse abdominus, external and internal obliques, spinalis, longissimus, ilicostalis, multifidi, rotatores, semispinalis capitis, intertransversarii, interspinalis	
Joint 5	Hip	LL: flexion BL: extension, medial rotation	LL: Rectus femoris, gluteus medius (anterior fibers), gluteus minimus, tensor fasciae latae, sartorius, psoas major, iliacus BL: biceps femoris, semitendinosus, semimembranosus, gluteus maximus and medius (posterior fibers), adductor magnus, adductor longus, adductor brevis, gracilis, pectineus, tensor fasciae latae	LL: gluteus maximus (lower fibers), gluteus medius (posterior fibers), biceps femoris, semitendinosus, semimembranosus
Joint 6	Knee	Extension	Vastus medialis, vastus lateralis, rectus femoris, vastus intermedius	Possibly gastrocnemius
Joint 7	Ankle	Dorsiflexion	Tibialis anterior, extensor digitorum longus, extensor hallucis longus	LL: possibly gastrocnemius, soleus

(TA = top arm; BA = bottom arm; BL = bottom leg; LL = lifted leg)

BOAT POSE: NAVASANA

Benefits
- Strengthens the abdominal region and the iliopsoas group, which in turn will help improve a flattened lumbar curve.

- Sit with your feet on the floor and in line with your buttock bones. Take hold of the back of your thighs and draw your sternum closer to the front of your thighs.
- Lengthen the spine and feel the crown of your head lifting upward.
- Draw your navel to your spine and lean back, raising your feet from the floor so that you are balancing on your sitting bones.
- Take a few breaths, while getting your balance. On your next exhalation, straighten both legs upward, keeping them stiff with your inner thighs locked together.

- Let go of your thighs and straighten your arms to shoulder height, with the palms facing each other.
- Your spine should remain straight—the tendency is to collapse the chest and lower back inward. If this starts to happen, take hold of your thighs and bend your legs.
- Gradually build up to holding the pose for between two and three minutes. Be aware that you should not be creating tension in your face, neck, or shoulders. Use the strength of the abdominals to keep the spine elevated.

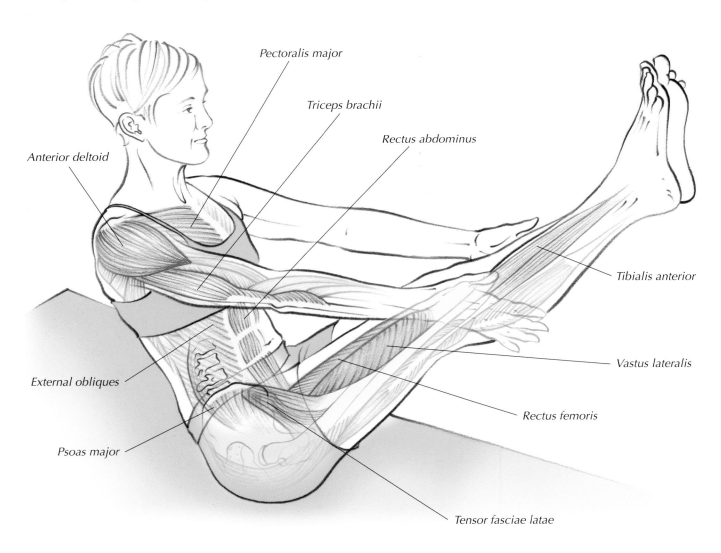

Pectoralis major

Triceps brachii

Rectus abdominus

Anterior deltoid

Tibialis anterior

Vastus lateralis

External obliques

Rectus femoris

Psoas major

Tensor fasciae latae

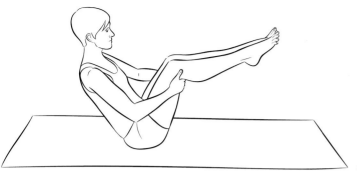

Modification 1
· If you find it easier to hold your legs, try not to do it for too long. Look to progress as soon as you can, keeping the spine elevated and the legs together.

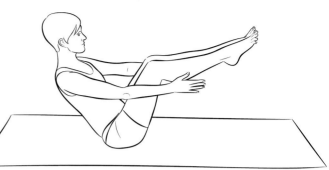

Modification 2
· Bending the legs with your arms on either side of your knees will help you build strength for the full pose.

ANALYSIS OF MOVEMENT	JOINTS	JOINT MOVEMENT	MUSCLES ACTIVE	MUSCLES STRETCHED
Joint 1	Scapula	Upward rotation, abduction	Trapezius (upper and lower fibers), serratus anterior, pectoralis minor	
Joint 2	Shoulder	Flexion, adduction, slight internal rotation	Anterior deltoid, pectoralis major, biceps brachii, coracobrachialis, infraspinatus, teres minor, posterior deltoid, latissimus dorsi, teres major	
Joint 3	Elbow	Extension	Triceps brachii, aconeus	
Joint 4	Spine	Neutral extension, resisting flexion	Spinalis, longissimus, ilicostalis, multifidi, rotatores, semispinalis capitis, intertransversarii, interspinalis, rectus abdominus, external and internal obliques, transverse abdominus	
Joint 5	Hip	Flexion, adduction, medial rotation	Rectus femoris, gluteus medius (anterior fibers), gluteus minimus, tensor fasciae latae, sartorius, psoas major, iliacus, adductor magnus, longus, and brevis, gracilis, pectineus, gluteus maximus (lower fibers)	Gluteus medius (posterior fibers), biceps femoris, semitendinosus, semimembranosus
Joint 6	Knee	Extension	Vastus medialis, lateralis, and intermedius, rectus femoris	Possibly gastrocnemius
Joint 7	Ankle	Dorsiflexion	Tibialis anterior, extensor digitorum longus, extensor hallucis longus	Possibly gastrocnemius, soleus

MOVING CATS: MARJARIASANA (VARIATION)

- Go onto all fours with your hands under your shoulders and your knees under your hips, drawing your navel in to your spine.
- As you inhale, straighten your right leg and lift it off the floor about 6–12 in. (15–30 cm) above the line of your buttock. Extend your heel away while keeping your pelvis straight and your hip bones in line. Direct your gaze to the floor.
- As you exhale, bend your right knee and draw it toward your forehead, bringing your forehead to your knee. Use your abdominals to bring your knee up as high as you can.
- Repeat this slowly as you breathe eight to twelve times on each side. To increase your strength, hold at the end of each movement for a few breaths.

Benefits
- Awakens and warms the thoracic and lumbar spine to flexion and extension. Also works to strengthen the iliopsoas group and the abdominals. This is an ideal posture to do first thing in the morning.

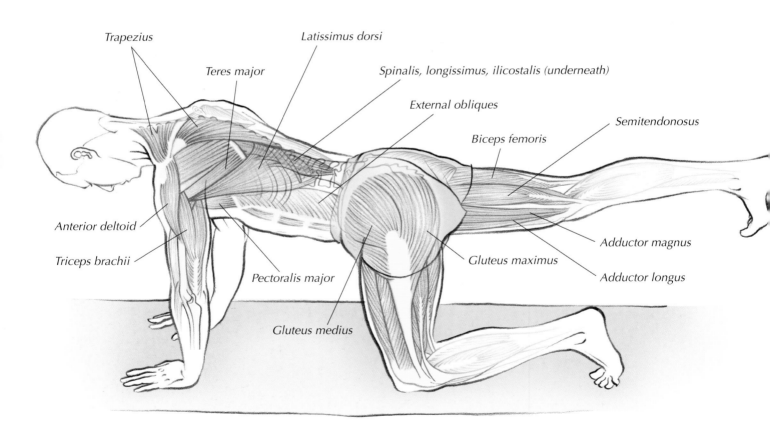

Trapezius

Latissimus dorsi

Teres major

Spinalis, longissimus, ilicostalis (underneath)

External obliques

Semitendonosus

Biceps femoris

Anterior deltoid

Triceps brachii

Adductor magnus

Gluteus maximus

Adductor longus

Pectoralis major

Gluteus medius

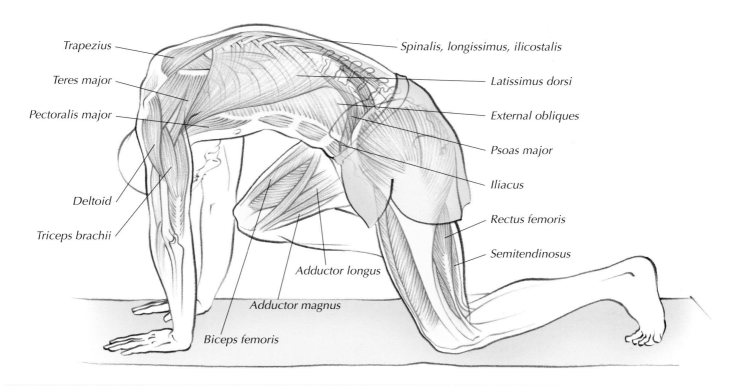

Trapezius
Teres major
Pectoralis major
Deltoid
Triceps brachii
Spinalis, longissimus, ilicostalis
Latissimus dorsi
External obliques
Psoas major
Iliacus
Rectus femoris
Semitendinosus
Adductor longus
Adductor magnus
Biceps femoris

ANALYSIS OF MOVEMENT	JOINTS	JOINT MOVEMENT	MUSCLES ACTIVE
Joint 1	Scapula	Upward rotation, abduction	Trapezius (upper and lower fibers), serratus anterior, pectoralis minor
Joint 2	Shoulder	Flexion, adduction, medial rotation	Anterior deltoid, pectoralis major, biceps brachii, coracobrachialis, latissimus dorsi, teres major, subscapularis
Joint 3	Elbow	Extension, pronation	Triceps brachii, aconeus, pronator teres, pronator quadratus, brachioradialis
Joint 4	Spine	Extension when lifted leg is straight, flexion when leg is bent	Spinalis, longissimus, ilicostalis, multifidi, rotatores, semispinalis capitis, intertransversarii, interspinalis, rectus abdominus, external and internal obliques, transverse abdominus
Joint 5	Hip	Leg extended, medially rotated	Biceps femoris, semitendinosus, semimembranosus, gluteus maximus, gluteus medius (posterior fibers), adductor magnus, adductor longus, adductor brevis, gracilis, pectineus, tensor fasciae latae
		Leg flexed, drawn into forehead	Rectus femoris, gluteus medius (anterior fibers), gluteus minimus, tensor fasciae latae, sartorius, psoas major, iliacus
		Stabilizing leg	Rectus femoris, gluteus medius (anterior fibers), gluteus minimus, tensor fasciae latae, sartorius, psoas major, iliacus
Joint 6	Knee	Knee extended	Vastus medialis, vastus lateralis, rectus femoris, vastus intermedius
		Knee flexed, drawn into forehead	Biceps femoris, semitendinosus, semimembranosus, gracilis, sartorius, gastrocnemius, popliteus
		Stabilizing knee	Vastus medialis, vastus lateralis, rectus femoris, vastus intermedius

COBRA – BHUJANGASANA

- Place your hands underneath your shoulders.
- Press the tops of your feet to the floor, including the tops of the little toes, to anchor your tailbone.
- Press from your hands and lead with your chest, lifting the upper body from the floor.
- Keep your hips and pubic bone on the floor.
- As you lift, keep your shoulder blades anchored and your elbows drawn into the outer edges of your rib cage.
- Try to maintain a smooth curve in your back and keep your gaze on the horizon or the floor. In this variation, the back of the neck maintains length; try not to push the chin forward.
- Lift as far as is comfortable, keeping your shoulders down and away from your ears and the pubic bone on the floor.
- Hold the pose for up to two minutes, maintaining a smooth, even, diaphragmatic breath throughout.

Note:
- It is important not to allow the gluteus maximus to do most of the work in this pose.
- Keep the shoulder blades moving down toward the sacrum. If you allow your shoulders to raise, you will create unnecessary tension in your neck.

Benefits
- This posture can give relief to those suffering from bulging lumbar disk complaints, as it can help encourage the disk to slide back into place.

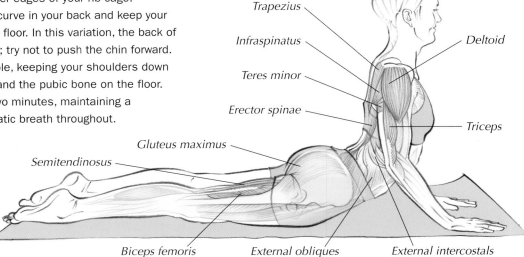

Trapezius · Infraspinatus · Teres minor · Erector spinae · Gluteus maximus · Semitendinosus · Deltoid · Triceps · Biceps femoris · External obliques · External intercostals

ANALYSIS OF MOVEMENT	JOINTS	JOINT MOVEMENT	MUSCLES ACTIVE	MUSCLES STRETCHED
Joint 1	Scapula	Depression	Trapezius (lower fibers), serratus anterior, pectoralis minor	
Joint 2	Shoulder	External rotation	Posterior deltoid, infraspinatus, teres minor	
Joint 3	Elbow	Extension, pronation	Triceps brachii, aconeus, pronator teres, pronator quadratus, brachioradialis	
Joint 4	Spine	Extension	Spinalis, longissimus, ilicostalis, multifidi, rotatores, semispinalis capitis, intertransversarii, interspinalis	Rectus abdominus, external and internal obliques, external intercostals
Joint 5	Hip	Extension, internal rotation, adduction	Biceps femoris, semitendinosus, semimembranosus, gluteus maximus, gluteus medius (anterior fibers), gluteus minimus, adductor magnus, adductor longus, adductor brevis, gracilis, pectineus, tensor fasciae latae	Possibly rectus femoris, psoas major, iliacus
Joint 6	Knee	Extension	Vastus medialis, vastus lateralis, rectus femoris, vastus intermedius	

LOCUST POSE 2: SHALABASANA (VARIATION)

- Lie face-down, straighten your legs, and press the tops of your feet lightly into the floor; your knees should lift.
- Place your arms alongside your body, with your palms to the floor. Rest your forehead on the floor.
- Draw your navel toward your spine, connecting with your core.
- Inhale, then slowly lift your chest, shoulders, hands, head, and legs from the floor. Turn your hands out so that your palms are facing away from your body. Keep the back of the neck long, gazing at the floor. Resist the urge to jut your chin forward and look up.

- Keep the length in the spine by allowing the crown of your head to keep moving forward, away from the sacrum.
- Maintain a smooth, even, diaphragmatic breath. Gradually build up to holding the pose for four minutes.

Benefits
- Strengthens both the lower and upper back muscles. Effective in increasing strength to draw the shoulders back and in improving postural imbalances. Also strengthens the buttock muscles. Can help poor digestion.

> ### Modification
> - Only lift your legs and upper body from the floor—keep your palms pressing to the floor and your anterior shoulders lifted.

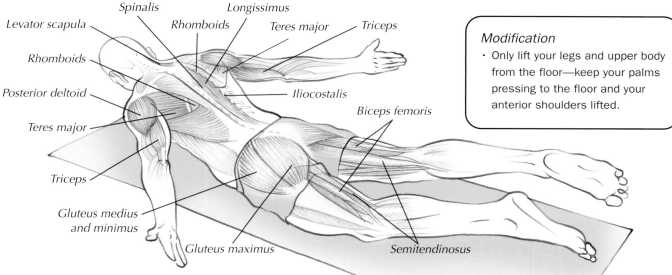

Spinalis · Longissimus · Rhomboids · Teres major · Triceps · Levator scapula · Rhomboids · Posterior deltoid · Iliocostalis · Teres major · Biceps femoris · Triceps · Gluteus medius and minimus · Gluteus maximus · Semitendinosus

ANALYSIS OF MOVEMENT	JOINTS	JOINT MOVEMENT	MUSCLES ACTIVE
Joint 1	Scapula	Downward rotation, adduction	Rhomboid major and minor, levator scapula
Joint 2	Shoulder	Extension, external rotation	Posterior deltoid, latissimus dorsi, teres major, subscapularis, pectoralis major, teres minor, infraspinatus, triceps brachii (long head)
Joint 3	Elbow	Extension, supination	Triceps brachii, aconeus, biceps brachii, supinator, brachioradialis
Joint 4	Spine	Extension	Spinalis, longissimus, ilicostalis, multifidi, rotatores, semispinalis capitis, intertransversarii, interspinalis
Joint 5	Hip	Extension, internal rotation, adduction	Biceps femoris, semitendinosus, semimembranosus, gluteus maximus, gluteus medius (anterior fibers), gluteus minimus, adductor magnus, longus, and brevis, gracilis, pectineus, tensor fasciae latae
Joint 6	Knee	Extension	Rectus femoris, vastus lateralis, medialis, and intermedius

RECLINING TWIST

Benefits
- Relieves tension and improves mobility in the lower back and hips. Frees the chest and shoulders. Improves digestion and elimination.

- Lie flat on your back and draw your heels toward your sitting bones (ischial tuberosities). Bring your arms to shoulder height, pointing your fingertips away. Turn your palms up and relax your shoulders.
- Lift your right leg and cross it over your left knee, the back of your right knee should connect with the top of your left knee.
- Inhale and lengthen the back of your neck.
- Exhale slowly and drop both knees to the left as far as is comfortable. As you inhale, settle into the stretch, breathing deeply into your abdomen and lower rib cage.
- Keep your right shoulder pressing to the floor and draw the right side of your rib cage to the floor.
- Remain in the pose for up to three minutes on each side. Direct the breath into the abdominal area to create a calming effect.
- When you are ready to come out of the pose, bring your knees back to the center on an exhalation, drawing your navel to your spine in order to use your abdominals to return your legs.

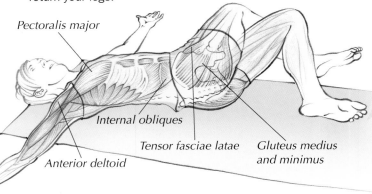

Pectoralis major
Internal obliques
Tensor fasciae latae
Gluteus medius and minimus
Anterior deltoid

ANALYSIS OF MOVEMENT	JOINTS	JOINT MOVEMENT	MUSCLES ACTIVE	MUSCLES STRETCHED
Joint 1	Scapula	Adduction	Trapezius (middle fibers), rhomboid major and minor	
Joint 2	Shoulder	Horizontal abduction, external rotation	Deltoid, subscapularis, teres minor, infraspinatus	Possibly anterior deltoid, pectoralis major of the shoulder opposite to the direction of the knees
Joint 3	Elbow	Extension, supination	Triceps brachii, aconeus, biceps brachii, supinator, brachioradialis	
Joint 4	Spine	Rotation	Multifidi, rotatores, external and internal obliques	Internal obliques of the stretched side
Joint 5	Hip	TL: flexion, adduction, internal rotation BL: flexion, abduction, external rotation	TL: rectus femoris, tensor fasciae latae, sartorius, psoas major, iliacus, adductor magnus, longus, and brevis, gracilis, pectineus, gluteus maximus (lower fibers), gluteus medius (anterior fibers), gluteus minimus BL: rectus femoris, gluteus medius (anterior fibers), gluteus minimus, tensor fasciae latae, sartorius, psoas major, iliacus, gluteus maximus, quadratus femoris, obturator internus and externus, gemellus superior and inferior	TL: possibly gluteus medius, gluteus minimus (lower fibers), tensor fasciae latae

(TL = top leg; BL = bottom leg)

CORPSE POSE: SAVASANA

"Sava" means corpse; this is a deep relaxation pose in which the body is motionless, appearing like a corpse. We spend most of our daily lives moving and not enjoying stillness—this is the time to experience deep stillness and inner calm.

Concentrate your mind on the subtle movements of your breath and the rise and fall of the abdomen. On each exhalation, have a sense of letting go of tension; allow the body to surrender to gravity. Try not to get caught up in unnecessary thoughts. Just allow the body to be.

- Start on your back with your heels toward the sitting bones, then gently straighten one leg at a time. Stretch your legs away from you. Draw your pubic bone toward you for a second, lengthening the lower back, then relax.
- Have the legs a little wider than hip-width apart. Straighten your arms away from your body, palms up, and relax your shoulders away from your ears. Lengthen your head away from your shoulders.
- Soften the skin of your face and let your jaw part slightly. Remain resting in this pose for between five and ten minutes.

- When you have finished, roll onto your right side, rest here for a few moments, and open your eyes. Gently bring yourself into a sitting position, becoming aware of your surroundings.
- If you find tension developing in your neck, place a small blanket underneath your neck to help keep it lengthened. You may also place a blanket underneath your knees to take any stress out of the lower back. An eyemask can be used on the eyes, as this is effective in calming the nervous system.

Benefits
- "Lying upon one's back on the ground at full length like a corpse removes fatigue caused by the other asana and induces calmness of mind" (S. Muktibodhananda, *Hatha Yoga Pradipika*). This posture gives the body time to relax and enjoy stillness and has a calming effect on the nervous system.

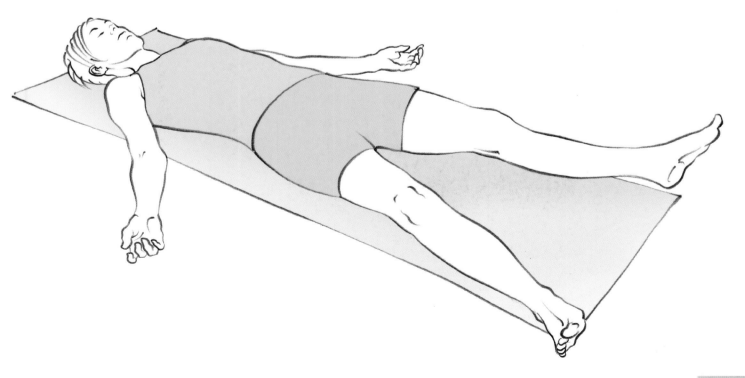

The marked changes in a flat-back posture are a reduced lumbar curve and an increased cervical spine, which is often referred to as "forward head." Due to the position of the head in relation to the torso, there is a likelihood of breathing difficulties. This could be mouth breathing or upper chest breathing. The following practice focuses on increasing the length of the breath, with a strong focus on the alignment of the head.

Three-part inhalation (viloma)

Come to a comfortable sitting position, using a block or a blanket to encourage an anterior tilt in the pelvis. Focus your attention on the position of your head. Bring your right hand up to your face and place two fingers on your chin. Gently press your chin backward toward your throat, allowing your head to move backward in line with your torso. You will feel the back of your neck lengthen. Allow the chin to drop slightly toward your sternum. Try not to force your head back, as this will eventually cause tension in your neck. When you are comfortable with the position, rest your hands on your knees in jnana mudra, palms down (see three-part exhalation on page 92 for a description of mudra).

Once you have found comfort in your sitting position, bring your awareness to your breathing. Try to make sure that your breath is moving through your nostrils and not your mouth. Relax every part of your body and scan your body with your mind from your feet, ankles, shins, and so on until you reach your head. As you reach your head, clarify your position, checking that you haven't moved your head forward. Relax your face and shoulders.

Begin the practice by inhaling for two seconds, then pause for two seconds holding the breath, inhale for two seconds, pause for two seconds holding the breath, inhale for two seconds, pause for two seconds holding the breath, then release the breath, exhaling through the nostrils. Exhale slowly and deeply, allowing it to last for a count of eight to ten. The last third of the breath will move right up into the rib crests.

It is important to maintain a softness in the shoulders and face. If you find that you are straining and feel uncomfortable, reduce the pauses to one second. During each pause, draw the navel to the spine and release it as you start the inhalation again. Stay conscious of the position of your head throughout the practice. Do not hold the pause for any longer than two seconds. Continue with this practice for ten to fifteen rounds.

Note:

If you suffer from high blood pressure, this practice should be done lying down.

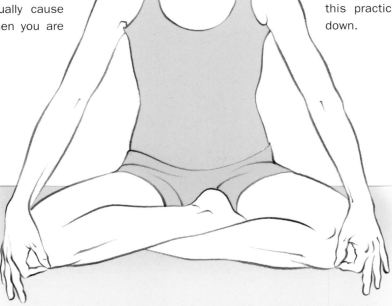

The phrase "antar mouna" is Sanskrit: antar meaning "inner" and mouna meaning "silence." A powerful meditation from the tantras (scriptures), it is normally a very in-depth practice that takes you deep into the realms of your mind in five stages, but for this particular practice we will be shortening it to just the first stage.

We spend a great deal of our daily lives with our minds focused on our external environment, with very little understanding of the events taking place within us. The purpose of antar mouna is to turn our attention toward our internal environment, creating a deep connection with our true essence. The practice will leave you feeling calm and present.

If you wish to learn more about the full five stages of this practice, it is advisable to seek a satyananda yoga teacher.

The practice

Come into a sitting posture, choosing one that you know you will feel comfortable in. We have used the kneeling pose for this practice, but if this is not comfortable, then choose one from the poses on page 38.

Settling yourself, take a deep breath through the nose and exhale through the mouth. Then allow your breathing to return to its natural pattern. Become aware of your body. With your full attention, become aware of the sensations and feelings that may arise. Feel the connection between your body and the floor, then move to your face. Notice the sensations around your eyes, mouth, and jaw, then move to your shoulders, arms, torso (both front and back), pelvis, upper legs, lower legs, ankles, feet, and toes.

Notice how your body moves with your breath. Let your body be as it is.

Notice that you can separate your awareness from your body, as if watching it. This is the ability to witness. It can take a while for you to tune into your body and for your mind to calm its thoughts.

Allow your awareness to run through the different parts of the body again, and be conscious of how the body feels. Pause for a minute before continuing.

Now start to notice the sounds around you, taking a little time to settle into listening. There is no need to identify what you hear, just witness the sounds that come to you. Start by becoming aware of the sounds closest to you, the softest sounds, then listen to the sounds in the distance and sounds from all directions. Pause for a moment, then come back to listening to the sounds that are closest. Focus on the beginning, middle, and end of the sound, even the faintest sounds.

Move your awareness to the taste in your mouth: are you able to taste your last meal, can you taste more on different areas of your tongue? Just notice. The sense of taste is always there.

Then focus on to the scents within your nose. Move away now to notice the smells surrounding you, focusing with all your awareness. Awaken your sensory muscles.

Finally, with your eyes closed, look forward into the space in front of your eyes. Look intently: notice the depth of your vision, how far you can see, notice colors inside your closed eyelids. Let your vision be as it is. Witness what arises.

Gently move your awareness back to the sounds around you, and with your eyes closed picture your surroundings. Take a few deep breaths, exhaling through your mouth. At this point, cultivate a sense of gratitude and love for all that surrounds you, then start to move slowly back into the world, opening your eyes and stretching.

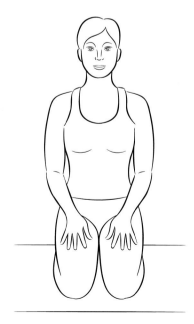

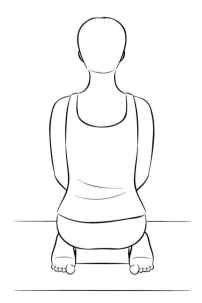

FLAT-BACK POSTURE

SWAY-BACK POSTURE

A sway-back posture (also known as "sway posture") is where the hips seen from the side sit forward of their normal position. A sway-back posture normally coincides with a decrease in lumbar curvature, especially in the lower lumbar area, and a posterior rotation of the pelvis. The hip joints can be extended or flexed.

The thoracic spine will compensate above it to maintain the center of gravity by increasing its kyphosis, with a posterior translation of the upper thoracic spine and forward movement of the head. The knees can hyperextend or flex.

With a sway-back posture, there will be a tightening of the hamstrings and the upper fibers of the internal obliques. There is also lengthening and weakening of the iliopsoas, external obliques, thoracic extensors, and neck flexors.

Physical causes

A sway-back posture is often caused by:

- A forward head posture—the pelvis shifts forward under the head in an attempt to maintain balance over the base of support
- An atlas subluxation, causing the head to move forward

Emotional causes

In the field of somatics, the sway-back posture represents a collapsed pattern, and a structure of this type can display weakness and fear (S. Keleman, *Emotional Anatomy*). A state of mind that may be experienced is that of disinterest; there may be a tendancy to fantasize frequently about how things could be different or one may be apathetic. The muscles that are active in maintaining an upright posture become heavy, drawing down toward the earth rather than lifting up, giving the internal sense of being unappreciated and resentful or helpless.

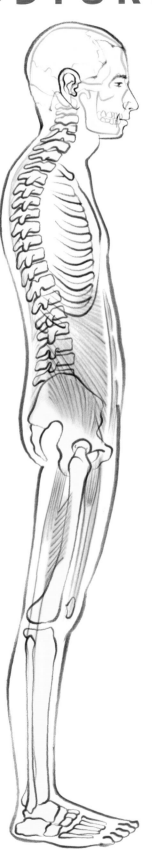

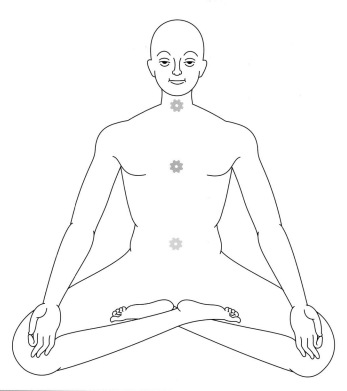

Forward head	Posterior pelvic tilt	Contracted chest	Rounded shoulders	Tight hamstrings
Encounter the world first with the head	Lessening of sexual energy and holding of sexual feelings	Underdeveloped ability to be self-expressive and self-assertive	Take on too many responsibilities	Related to self-control issues
	Inability to stay grounded in emotional activity	Feelings of insecurity	Feelings of being overburdened by life itself	Difficulty in letting go
	Feelings are constricted or constrained	Will be more passive than aggressive		Fears of being abandoned
		More motivated by a chronic sense of fear and inferiority		Fears of loss of support

Chakra	Positive feelings cultivated	Location	Bija mantra
Solar plexus chakra/ 3rd—manipura	Self-confidence Courage Fearless of life's challenges	The part of the vertebral column that relates to the navel; solar plexus	Ram
Heart chakra/4th—anahata	Compassion Unconditional love Forgiveness for oneself and others	The part of the vertebral column that relates to the heart; cardiac plexus	Yam
Throat chakra/5th—vishuddha	Truthful speech Honesty to oneself Freedom of self-expression	The neck region; the cervical part of the spinal column, related to the throat; carotid plexus	Ham

DOWN DOG: ADHO MUKHA SHVANASANA

- Come into a kneeling position with your buttocks to your heels, then fold forward, taking your head down to the floor, and push your arms forward as far as possible, shoulder-width apart.
- As you inhale, bring yourself up on all fours, keeping your hands where they are. You will find that your shoulders are slightly behind your hands: this is the perfect position.
- Slightly lift your sitting bones, creating a slight anterior tilt to your pelvis.
- As you exhale, maintain the anterior tilt, lifting your sitting bones up and away from your hands, resembling a pyramid.

- Press both hands down and forward into the mat, especially the thumb and index finger base, not gripping with your fingers. As you press down, lift your shoulders away.
- Press your front thighs back into your hamstrings, and your shins into your calves. Slightly roll your thighs inward, broadening across the buttocks.
- Press your inner and outer heels evenly into the floor as you simultaneously lift your sitting bones, creating a two-way stretch.
- Roll the biceps upward to create space between your shoulders and ears. Soften your neck, allowing your ears to stay in the same line as your upper arms and resist the urge to look forward or look up underneath you.
- Remain in the pose for up to two minutes. Maintain an even, diaphragmatic breath.

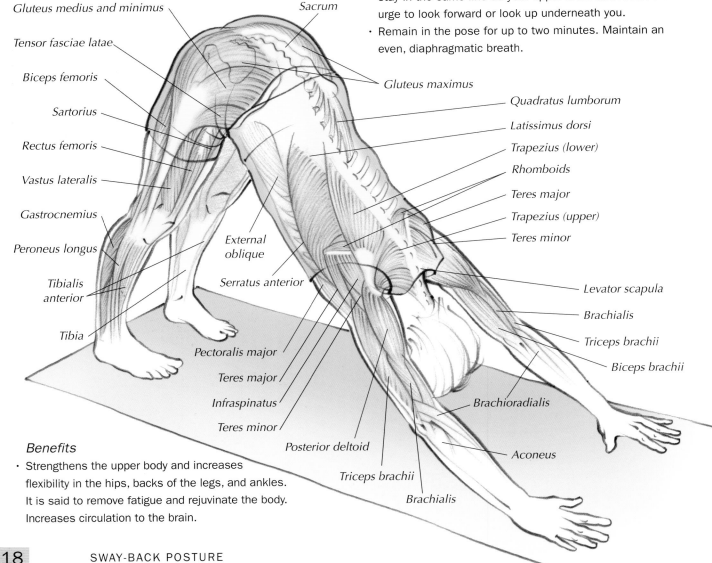

Gluteus medius and minimus

Tensor fasciae latae

Biceps femoris

Sartorius

Rectus femoris

Vastus lateralis

Gastrocnemius

Peroneus longus

Tibialis anterior

Tibia

External oblique

Serratus anterior

Pectoralis major

Teres major

Infraspinatus

Teres minor

Posterior deltoid

Triceps brachii

Brachialis

Sacrum

Gluteus maximus

Quadratus lumborum

Latissimus dorsi

Trapezius (lower)

Rhomboids

Teres major

Trapezius (upper)

Teres minor

Levator scapula

Brachialis

Triceps brachii

Biceps brachii

Brachioradialis

Aconeus

Benefits
- Strengthens the upper body and increases flexibility in the hips, backs of the legs, and ankles. It is said to remove fatigue and rejuvinate the body. Increases circulation to the brain.

118   SWAY-BACK POSTURE

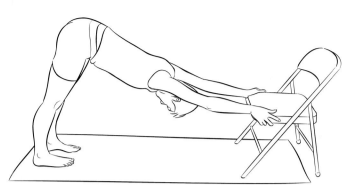

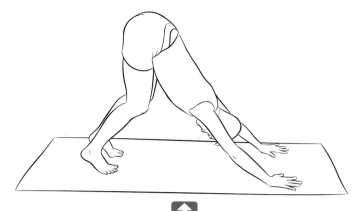

Modification 1
- A chair can help take the weight of your upper body when you first start. It will also encourage the two-way stretch in the back of the legs.

Modification 2
- Bending the knees will also reduce the stretch in the back of the knees and help you maintain the pelvis in an anterior tilt.

ANALYSIS OF MOVEMENT	JOINTS	JOINT MOVEMENT	MUSCLES ACTIVE	MUSCLES STRETCHED
Joint 1	Scapula	Upward rotation, elevation	Trapezius (upper and lower fibers), rhomboid major and minor, levator scapula	
Joint 2	Shoulder	Flexion, external rotation, abduction	Posterior and anterior deltoid, pectoralis major (upper fibers), biceps brachii, coracobrachialis, infraspinatus, teres minor, serratus anterior, pectoralis minor	Teres minor, latissimus dorsi
Joint 3	Elbow	Extension, pronation	Triceps brachii, aconeus, pronator teres, pronator quadratus, brachioradialis	
Joint 4	Spine	Extension	Spinalis, longissimus, ilicostalis, multifidi, rotatores, semispinalis capitis, intertransversarii, interspinalis	
Joint 5	Hip	Flexion, internal rotation	The intention is not to have the deep hip flexors active, but will activate adductor magnus, adductor longus, adductor brevis, gracilis	Gluteus maximus
Joint 6	Knee	Extension	Rectus femoris, vastus lateralis, vastus medialis, vastus intermedius	Biceps femoris, semitendinosus, semimembranosus
Joint 7	Ankle	Dorsiflexion	Tibialis anterior, extensor digitorum longus, extensor hallucis longus	Gastrocnemius, soleus, plantaris

HALF SPLITS: ARDHA HANUMANASANA

Starting position ➡️

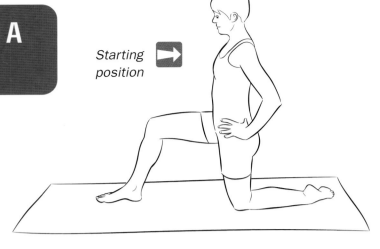

- Come to an upright kneeling position, then lunge your left foot forward. Bring the leg to a 90 degree angle, then shift your foot forward about another length of your foot.
- Keep your left hip directly over your left knee.
- As you exhale, bend forward at your hips and place your hands on either side of your left leg. Keep your left foot flat to begin with, keeping a bend in that knee.
- Press the left heel away and into the floor, and lift your sitting bones upward and your tailbone backward, creating a two-way movement in the back of your left leg.
- Try to achieve an anterior tilt of your pelvis.

- Stay in this position for several breaths. If you wish to take this further, you can pivot your foot onto the heel and straighten your left leg, still keeping the two-way stretch.

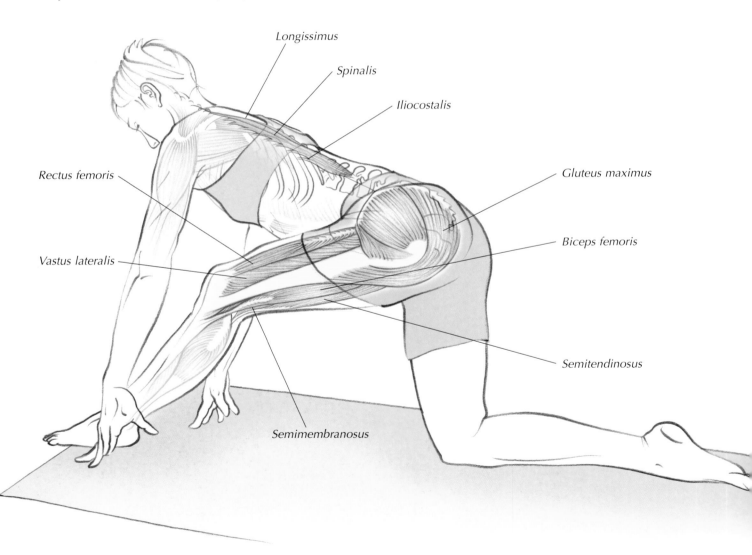

Longissimus

Spinalis

Iliocostalis

Gluteus maximus

Rectus femoris

Biceps femoris

Vastus lateralis

Semitendinosus

Semimembranosus

- Maintain extension through the thoracic spine, making sure not to collapse forward over your leg. Keep the back of your neck lengthened without dropping your forehead toward your leg.
- Remain in the pose for between two and three minutes, maintaining a smooth, even, diaphragmatic breath.
- Come out of the pose slowly by bringing your left leg back to join your right. Rest in an all-fours position before completing the asana on the opposite side.

Benefits
- Effective in stretching the hamstrings. Can aid digestion.

Modification
- The use of blocks can help maintain extension in the spine and lift in the sitting bones. A chair can also be used, by resting your hands on a chair in front of you.

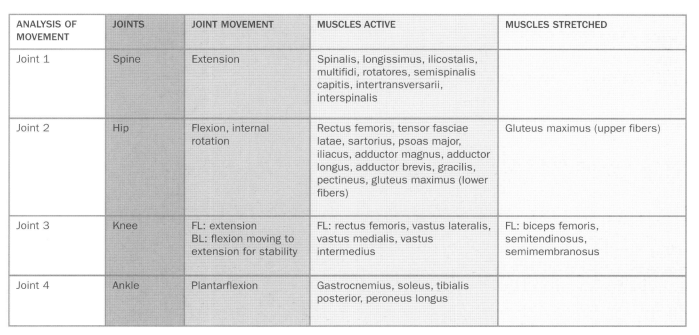

ANALYSIS OF MOVEMENT	JOINTS	JOINT MOVEMENT	MUSCLES ACTIVE	MUSCLES STRETCHED
Joint 1	Spine	Extension	Spinalis, longissimus, ilicostalis, multifidi, rotatores, semispinalis capitis, intertransversarii, interspinalis	
Joint 2	Hip	Flexion, internal rotation	Rectus femoris, tensor fasciae latae, sartorius, psoas major, iliacus, adductor magnus, adductor longus, adductor brevis, gracilis, pectineus, gluteus maximus (lower fibers)	Gluteus maximus (upper fibers)
Joint 3	Knee	FL: extension BL: flexion moving to extension for stability	FL: rectus femoris, vastus lateralis, vastus medialis, vastus intermedius	FL: biceps femoris, semitendinosus, semimembranosus
Joint 4	Ankle	Plantarflexion	Gastrocnemius, soleus, tibialis posterior, peroneus longus	

(FL = front leg; BL = back leg)

TRIANGLE POSE: UTTITHA TRIKONASANA (VARIATION)

Starting position ➡

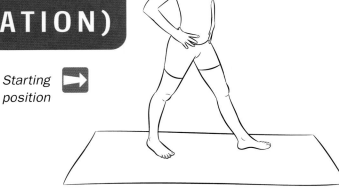

- Stand with your feet 3 ft. (1 m) apart, with your hands on your hips.
- Turn your left foot out 90 degrees by pivoting on your heel and lifting your toes. Pivot your right foot about 60 degrees by lifting your heel up from the floor and moving it toward the short edge of the mat (see starting position illustration).
- Press your left heel down as if you are attempting to increase the weight on a scale. Your left outer hip should move backward as your right frontal hip bone moves slightly forward. Do not hyperextend your front knee.
- Maintain the action in your left leg as you press the outer heel of your right foot firmly into the ground. In turn, roll the upper inner right thigh backward.
- Inhale and reach your left arm forward, allowing your torso to follow, and then lower it to the floor so that your fingertips are in line with your shin or ankle. Your torso should now be parallel to the floor.
- Exhale and draw the navel to the spine and draw the tailbone inward.
- Inhale slowly and reach your right arm upward, opening your chest. Keep your gaze toward your fingertips.

- Focus on keeping strength throughout your torso by drawing the navel to the spine. Lift the rib cage away from the pelvis so that you are not collapsing the left side of your torso.
- Maintain a steady diaphragmatic breath, with a relaxed face and jaw.
- Remain in the pose for between two and three minutes. Come out of the asana with an inhalation.

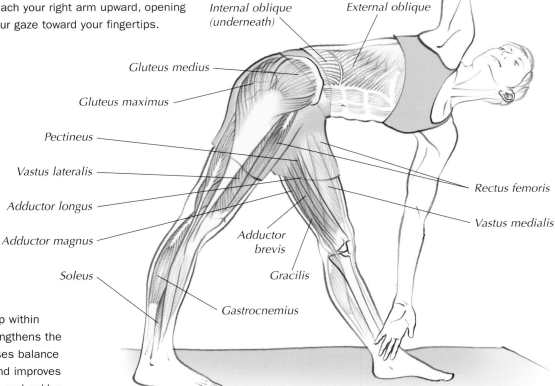

Internal oblique (underneath)

External oblique

Gluteus medius

Gluteus maximus

Pectineus

Vastus lateralis

Adductor longus

Adductor magnus

Soleus

Adductor brevis

Gracilis

Gastrocnemius

Rectus femoris

Vastus medialis

Benefits
- Builds strength deep within the spine. Also strengthens the abdominals, increases balance and coordination, and improves flexibility in the hips and ankles.

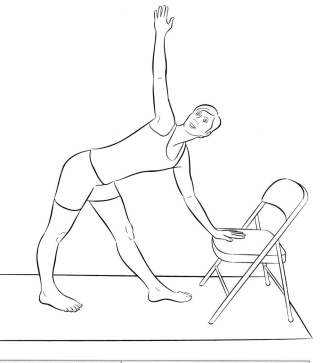

Note:

- The triangle pose is a classical asana. For the purpose of this particular practice, the alignment has been altered. The approach taken in this text is to reduce unnecessary loading on the sacro-iliac joint.

Modification

- As with the previous asana, use a chair until you build strength and flexibility. The chair gives support, which enables you to learn the alignment.

ANALYSIS OF MOVEMENT	JOINTS	JOINT MOVEMENT	MUSCLES ACTIVE	MUSCLES STRETCHED
Joint 1	Spine	Extension, rotation	Spinalis, longissimus, ilicostalis, multifidi, rotatores, semispinalis capitis, intertransversarii, interspinalis, external and internal obliques	
Joint 2	Hip	FL: flexion, external rotation BL: flexion, internal rotation	FL: rectus femoris, tensor fasciae latae, sartorius, psoas major, iliacus, biceps femoris, gluteus maximus, gluteus medius (posterior fibers), piriformis, quadratus femoris, obturator internus, obturator externus, gemellus superior, gemellus inferior BL: rectus femoris, tensor fasciae latae, sartorius, psoas major, iliacus, adductor magnus, adductor longus, adductor brevis, gracilis, pectineus, gluteus maximus (lower fibers)	FL: adductor magnus, adductor longus, adductor brevis, gracilis, pectineus, semimembranosus, semitendinosus, biceps femoris BL: gluteus maximus, gluteus medius (posterior fibers), piriformis, sartorius, quadratus femoris, obturator internus, obturator externus, gemellus superior, gemellus inferior
Joint 3	Knee	Extension	Rectus femoris, vastus lateralis, vastus medialis, vastus intermedius	
Joint 4	Ankle	FL: plantarflexion, slight pronation BL: dorsiflexion, slight pronation	FL: gastrocnemius, soleus, tibialis posterior, peroneus longus, peroneus brevis, extensor digitorum longus BL: tibialis anterior, extensor digitorum longus, extensor hallucis longus	

(FL = front leg; BL = back leg)

REVOLVED TRIANGLE POSE: PARIVRTTA TRIKONASANA (VARIATION)

- Stand with your feet one-leg's distance apart and turn your left foot 90 degrees by pivoting on your left heel and your back foot 60 degrees by lifting onto the toe and pivoting the heel outward from the left heel.
- Turn your hips, torso, chest, and shoulders to face your left leg.
- Press your left foot down and forward into the floor, grounding the inner edge of the foot.
- Press your right heel deeply into the floor and backward, grounding the outer edge of the foot. Try to bring both frontal pelvic bones into the same plane.
- Keep both legs straight. By pressing firmly through your front foot, you will prevent hyperextension in your front knee.
- As you inhale, reach forward with your right arm, bringing your torso parallel to the floor. Try to keep the sacrum flat.

- Exhale and move your right hand to the outside of your left foot.
- Keep both sides of your waist lengthened and your sitting bones lifted. Inhale and lift your left arm upward, opening your chest to the left. Turn your gaze to your left thumb.
- As your left foot presses down and forward, keep your outer left hip moving backward, creating length along the left side of the torso.
- Your feet should stay firmly grounded.
- Gradually build up to holding the pose for up to three minutes on each side.
- When you come out of the posture, draw your navel in, inhale, and lead up with your right arm, keeping both legs straight.

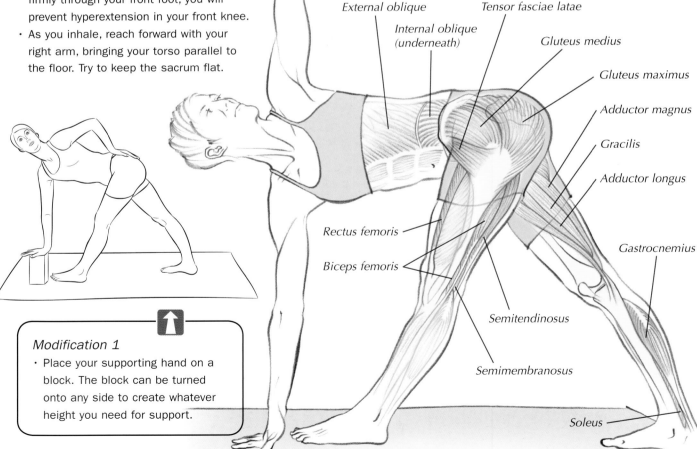

External oblique
Internal oblique (underneath)
Tensor fasciae latae
Gluteus medius
Gluteus maximus
Adductor magnus
Gracilis
Adductor longus
Rectus femoris
Biceps femoris
Gastrocnemius
Semitendinosus
Semimembranosus
Soleus

Modification 1
- Place your supporting hand on a block. The block can be turned onto any side to create whatever height you need for support.

Benefits
- Aids digestion and internal organ motility. Increases flexibility in the hips and improves rotational mobility in the spine.

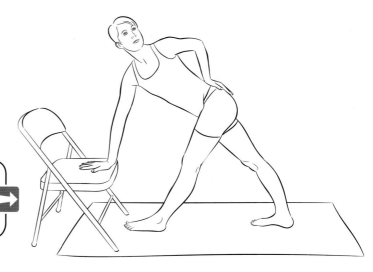

Modification 2
- The use of a chair is a good starting place if your hamstrings are especially short.

ANALYSIS OF MOVEMENT	JOINTS	JOINT MOVEMENT	MUSCLES ACTIVE	MUSCLES STRETCHED
Joint 1	Scapula	Adduction	Trapezius (middle fibers), rhomboid major and minor	
Joint 2	Shoulder	Horizontal abduction, external rotation	Deltoid, subscapularis, teres minor, infraspinatus, supraspinatus	Latissimus dorsi, teres major
Joint 3	Spine	Extension, rotation	Spinalis, longissimus, ilicostalis, multifidi, rotatores, semispinalis capitis, intertransversarii, interspinalis, external and internal obliques	
Joint 4	Hip	FL: flexion, external rotation BL: flexion, internal rotation	FL: rectus femoris, tensor fasciae latae, sartorius, psoas major, iliacus, biceps femoris, gluteus maximus, gluteus medius (posterior fibers), piriformis, quadratus femoris, obturator internus, obturator externus, gemellus superior, gemellus inferior BL: rectus femoris, tensor fasciae latae, sartorius, psoas major, iliacus, adductor magnus, adductor longus, adductor brevis, gracilis, pectineus, gluteus maximus (lower fibers)	FL: adductor magnus, adductor longus, adductor brevis, gracilis, pectineus, semimembranosus, semitendinosus, biceps femoris BL: gluteus maximus, gluteus medius (posterior fibers), piriformis, sartorius, quadratus femoris, obturator internus, obturator externus, gemellus superior, gemellus inferior
Joint 5	Knee	Extension	Rectus femoris, vastus lateralis, vastus medialis, vastus intermedius	
Joint 6	Ankle	FL: plantarflexion, slight pronation BL: dorsiflexion, slight pronation	FL: gastrocnemius, soleus, tibialis posterior, peroneus longus, peroneus brevis, extensor digitorum longus BL: tibialis anterior, extensor digitorum longus, extensor hallucis longus	

(FL = front leg; BL = back leg)

GATE POSE: PARIGRASANA

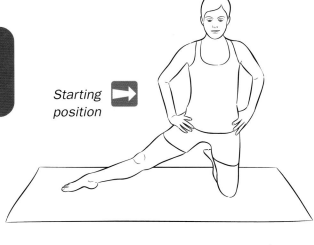

Starting position ➡️

- Kneel on the floor with your ankles together and your hips over your knees.
- Stretch your right leg out sideways to the right, keeping it in line with your left hip and trunk.
- Turn your right foot sideways so that it is pointing away from you. Keep your right leg straight.
- Look at your pelvis and align both of the frontal pelvic bones. Ensure that your left buttock is directly over your left knee.
- Imagine that your torso is in between two panes of glass.
- Put your right hand, with your palm facing up, on top of your right thigh.
- Inhale, lift your left arm, and reach your fingertips away from the floor, lengthening the left side of your body.
- Exhale and gently reach over to the right side as your right hand moves down the right thigh to your shin.

- Keep the left shoulder rolled back to prevent you from collapsing forward.
- The shoulders should be moving away from your ears, preventing uneccessary tension. Your gaze should remain forward.
- Remain in the pose for between two and three minutes, all the while lifting out of the pelvis and extending over your right leg.
- Maintain a smooth, even, diaphragmatic breath throughout the pose.
- Come out of the pose on an inhalation. Return to kneeling and remain resting in this position before repeating the pose on the opposite side.

Benefits
- Increases flexibility laterally to the torso and strengthens the internal and external obliques.

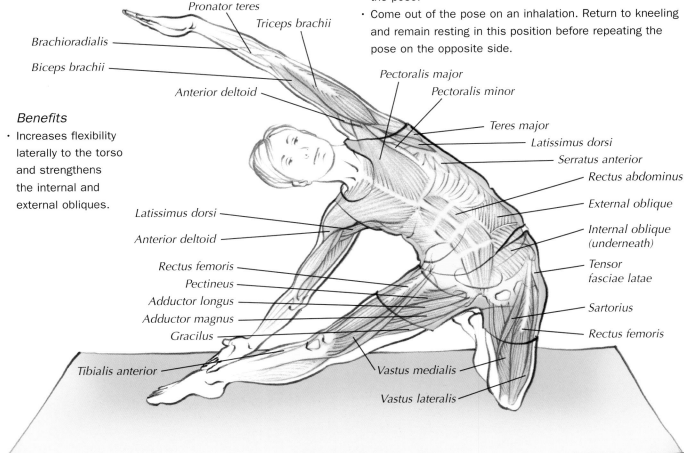

Pronator teres

Triceps brachii

Brachioradialis

Biceps brachii

Anterior deltoid

Pectoralis major

Pectoralis minor

Teres major

Latissimus dorsi

Serratus anterior

Rectus abdominus

External oblique

Internal oblique (underneath)

Latissimus dorsi

Anterior deltoid

Tensor fasciae latae

Rectus femoris

Pectineus

Adductor longus

Adductor magnus

Gracilus

Sartorius

Rectus femoris

Tibialis anterior

Vastus medialis

Vastus lateralis

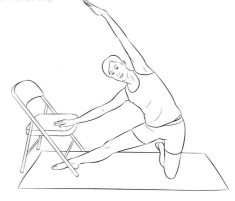

Modification

· The use of a chair will reduce the stretch in the upper side and will also help you build strength for the full asana. It can also help if you bend the straight leg—this will reduce the stretch in the hamstrings and adductors.

ANALYSIS OF MOVEMENT	JOINTS	JOINT MOVEMENT	MUSCLES ACTIVE	MUSCLES STRETCHED
Joint 1	Scapula	TA: upward rotation, abduction BA: neutral	TA: trapezius (upper and lower fibers), serratus anterior, pectoralis minor	Rhomboid major and minor
Joint 2	Shoulder	TA: abduction, external rotation, flexion BA: external rotation, abduction	TA: deltoid, infraspinatus, teres minor, pectoralis major (upper fibers), biceps brachii, coracobrachialis, supraspinatus BA: deltoid, infraspinatus, teres minor, pectoralis major (upper fibers)	Latissimus dorsi, triceps brachii (long head), teres major
Joint 3	Elbow	Extension, supination	Triceps brachii, aconeus, biceps brachii, supinator, brachioradialis	
Joint 4	Spine	Lateral flexion	External and internal obliques	
Joint 5	Hip	SL: neutral extension, adduction, internal rotation EL: flexion, external rotation, abduction	SL: semitendinosus, semimembranosus, gluteus medius (anterior fibers), gluteus minimus, adductor longus, adductor brevis, gracilis, pectineus, tensor fasciae latae, psoas major, iliacus EL: rectus femoris, tensor fasciae latae, sartorius, psoas major, iliacus, biceps femoris, gluteus maximus, gluteus medius (posterior fibers), piriformis, quadratus femoris, obturator internus, obturator externus, gemellus superior, gemellus inferior	EL: adductor magnus, adductor longus, adductor brevis, gracilis, pectineus, semimembranosus, semitendinosus, biceps femoris
Joint 6	Knee	SL: flexion moving to extension to stabilize EL: extension	SL: rectus femoris, vastus lateralis, vastus medialis, vastus intermedius EL: rectus femoris, vastus lateralis, vastus medialis, vastus intermedius	
Joint 7	Ankle	SL: dorsiflexion EL: plantarflexion	SL: tibialis anterior, extensor digitorum longus, extensor hallucis longus EL: gastrocnemius, soleus, tibialis posterior, peroneus longus	

(TA = top arm; BA = bottom arm; SL = supporting leg; EL = extended leg)

SEATED FORWARD BEND: PASCIMOTTANASANA (VARIATION)

- Sit with your legs outstretched, bring your inner thighs together, and flex your feet, extending through your inner heels.
- Take your arms behind you and use your hands to pivot onto the front of your sitting bones.
- Press the back of your thighs into the floor and continue extending your heels away from you.
- Inhale and lift your arms until they are vertical. As you exhale, pivot forward at your hips, moving your hands to hold onto the outer edges of your feet.
- Draw your chin slightly in toward your throat, extending the back of the neck. Imagine the crown of your head being drawn upward and slightly forward.
- Maintain a smooth, even, diaphragmatic breath for up to three minutes.
- With each inhalation extend the spine upward, keeping the shoulder blades moving back and the chest moving forward and up.
- It is important to maintain length in the spine—try not to collapse forward, creating an excessive thoracic curve.

Benefits
- In the traditional asana, the torso folds flat onto the knees. For the purpose of this practice, it is ideal to keep as much extension as possible in the spine. This will create a more effective stretch on the hamstrings. This posture also has a calming effect on the nervous system and aids digestion.

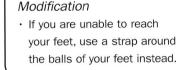

Modification
- If you are unable to reach your feet, use a strap around the balls of your feet instead.

Longissimus
Iliocostalis
Spinalis
Gluteus maximus
Piriformis
Glemellus superior
Oburator internus
Glemellus inferior
Biceps femoris
Oburator externus
Quadratus femoris major

ANALYSIS OF MOVEMENT	JOINTS	JOINT MOVEMENT	MUSCLES ACTIVE	MUSCLES STRETCHED
Joint 1	Spine	Flexion moving toward extension	Spinalis, longissimus, ilicostalis, multifidi, rotatores, semispinalis capitis, intertransversarii, interspinalis	
Joint 2	Hip	Flexion, adduction, internal rotation	Adductor magnus, longus and brevis, pectineus, gracilis, psoas major, iliacus, sartorius, gluteus maximus (lower fibers), gluteus medius (anterior fibers), gluteus minimus	Gluteus maximus (upper fibers), piriformis, quadratus femoris, obturator internus and externus, gemellus superior and inferior, gluteus medius (posterior fibers)
Joint 3	Knee	Extension	Rectus femoris, vastus lateralis, medialis and intermedius	Biceps femoris, semitendinosus, semimembranosus, gracilis, sartorius

BOAT POSE: NAVASANA

Modification
- If you find it easier to hold your legs, try not to do it for too long. Look to progress as soon as you can, keeping the spine elevated and the legs together.

- Sit with your feet on the floor and in line with your buttock bones. Take hold of the back of your thighs and draw your sternum closer to the front of your thighs.
- Lengthen the spine, feeling the crown of your head lifting upward.
- Draw your navel in to your spine, then lean back, taking your feet from the floor so that you are balancing on your sitting bones.
- Take a few breaths, getting your balance. On your next exhalation, straighten both legs upward and keep them stiff, with the inner thighs locked together.
- Let go of your thighs and straighten your arms to shoulder height, with your palms facing each other.
- Your spine should remain straight. The tendency is to collapse in the chest and lower back; if this starts to happen, take hold of your thighs and bend your legs.
- Gradually build up to holding the pose for up to three minutes. Be conscious that you are not creating tension in your face, neck, or shoulders. Use the strength of your abdominals to keep your spine elevated.

Benefits
- Strengthens the abdominal region and the iliopsoas group, which in turn will help improve a flattened lumbar curve.

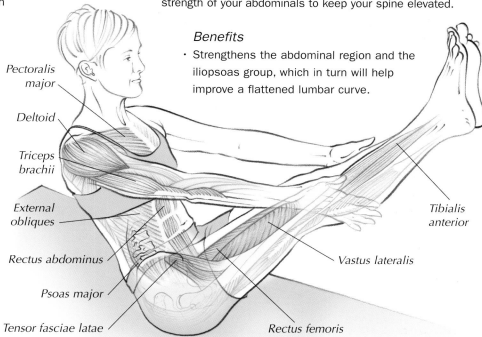

Pectoralis major

Deltoid

Triceps brachii

External obliques

Rectus abdominus

Psoas major

Tensor fasciae latae

Tibialis anterior

Vastus lateralis

Rectus femoris

ANALYSIS OF MOVEMENT	JOINTS	JOINT MOVEMENT	MUSCLES ACTIVE
Joint 1	Scapula	Upward rotation, abduction	Trapezius (upper and lower fibers), serratus anterior, pectoralis minor
Joint 2	Shoulder	Flexion, adduction, slight internal rotation	Anterior deltoid, pectoralis major, biceps brachii, coracobrachialis, infraspinatus, teres minor, posterior deltoid, latissimus dorsi, teres major
Joint 3	Elbow	Extension	Triceps brachii, aconeus
Joint 4	Spine	Neutral extension resisting flexion	Spinalis, longissimus, ilicostalis, multifidi, rotatores, semispinalis capitis, intertransversarii, interspinalis, rectus abdominus, external and internal obliques, transverse abdominus
Joint 5	Hip	Flexion, adduction, medial rotation	Rectus femoris, gluteus medius (anterior fibers), gluteus minimus, tensor fasciae latae, sartorius, psoas major, iliacus, adductor magnus, longus, and brevis, gracilis, pectineus, gluteus maximus (lower fibers)
Joint 6	Knee	Extension	Vastus medialis, lateralis, and intermedius, rectus femoris
Joint 7	Ankle	Dorsiflexion	Tibialis anterior, extensor digitorum longus, extensor hallucis longus

SIDE PLANK: VASISTHASANA

- Come into "down dog" and, as you inhale, shift your weight forward so that your shoulders are over your wrists.
- Exhale, shift your weight onto your right hand, and simultaneously turn onto the outer edge of your left foot. Move your right foot to rest on the inner edge of your left foot.
- Inhale and take your right arm up so that it comes in line with the right shoulder.
- Your body should be in one straight line. Align the center of your palm with the arch of your back foot.
- Lock your thighs together and straighten your legs, pressing your inner thighs together.
- Gradually build up to holding the pose for three minutes on each side.
- Be conscious not to create tension in your jaw or face—soften your jaw to relax your face.

Triceps brachii
Pectoralis major
Deltoid
Latissimus dorsi
Rectus abdominus
External obliques
Vastus lateralis
Rectus femoris
Tibialis anterior
Deltoid
Teres minor
Teres major
Triceps brachii
Gluteus medius and minimus
Vastus lateralis
Rectus femoris
Vastus medialis

Modification
- If you have wrist problems, resting your weight on your forearm will work better for you.
- If you find it difficult to balance, take the top foot forward onto the floor in line with the bottom foot.

Benefits
- Increases strength in the abdominals, arms, and hips.

ANALYSIS OF MOVEMENT	JOINTS	JOINT MOVEMENT	MUSCLES ACTIVE
Joint 1	Scapula	Downward rotation, adduction	Trapezius (middle fibers), rhomboid major and minor, levator scapula
Joint 2	Shoulder	Horizontal abduction, external rotation	Deltoid, supraspinatus, teres minor, infraspinatus, triceps brachii (long head)
Joint 3	Elbow	BA: extension, pronation TA: extension, neutral	BA: triceps brachii, aconeus, pronator teres, pronator quadratus TA: triceps brachii, aconeus
Joint 4	Spine	Neutral but active	Spinalis, longissimus, ilicostalis, multifidi, rotatores, semispinalis capitis, intertransversarii, interspinalis, rectus abdominus, transverse abdominus, external and internal obliques
Joint 5	Hip	Neutral extension, adduction, internal rotation	Rectus femoris, gluteus medius (anterior fibers), gluteus minimus, adductor magnus, longus, and brevis, pectineus, tensor fasciae latae, sartorius, psoas major, iliacus, gracilis, semitendinosus, semimembranosus, biceps femoris
Joint 6	Knee	Extension	Rectus femoris, vastus lateralis, medialis, and intermedius

(BA = bottom arm; TA = top arm)

LOCUST POSE 3: SHALABASANA (VARIATION)

Benefits
- Strengthens the lower and upper back muscles, improves postural imbalances and also strengthens buttock muscles. Can help poor digestion.

- Lie face-down, lengthen your legs away from you, and press the tops of your feet lightly into the floor, lifting your knees.
- Stretch your arms forward, taking them to a 45-degree angle. Turn your thumbs up, so that you are resting on the outer edges of your hands.
- Anchor the lowest point of your shoulder blades, creating space between your shoulders and your ears.
- Draw your navel toward your spine, connecting with your core.
- Inhale, then slowly lift your chest, arms, head, and legs from the floor so that only your pelvis stays grounded. Keep the back of your neck long and your gaze on the floor. Resist the urge to jut your chin forward and look up.
- Open across your chest and reach forward to your fingertips.

- Point your toes away from your hips and have your legs no wider than hip-width apart.
- Keep the length in the spine by allowing the crown of your head to keep moving forward, away from the sacrum.
- Gradually build up to holding the pose for four minutes, maintaining an even diaphragmatic breath throughout. Keep your face and jaw soft.

Modifications
- Keep the legs and feet on the floor and just lift the upper body.
- See locust pose 2 on page 112.

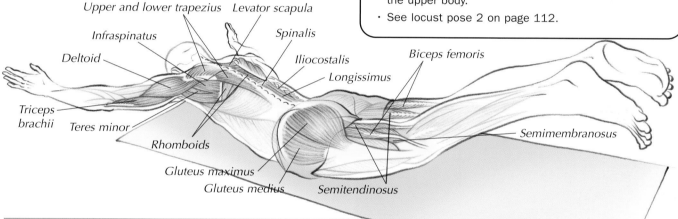

Upper and lower trapezius • Levator scapula • Spinalis • Iliocostalis • Longissimus • Infraspinatus • Deltoid • Biceps femoris • Triceps brachii • Teres minor • Rhomboids • Gluteus maximus • Gluteus medius • Semitendinosus • Semimembranosus

ANALYSIS OF MOVEMENT	JOINTS	JOINT MOVEMENT	MUSCLES ACTIVE
Joint 1	Scapula	Upward rotation, elevation	Trapezius (upper and lower fibers), rhomboid major and minor, levator scapula
Joint 2	Shoulder	Flexion, external rotation	Deltoid (posterior fibers), pectoralis major (upper fibers), teres minor, infraspinatus, biceps brachii, coracobrachialis
Joint 3	Elbow	Extension, supination	Triceps brachii, aconeus, biceps brachii, supinator, brachioradialis
Joint 4	Spine	Extension	Spinalis, longissimus, ilicostalis, multifidi, rotatores, semispinalis capitis, intertransversarii, interspinalis
Joint 5	Hip	Extension, internal rotation, adduction	Biceps femoris, semitendinosus, semimembranosus, gluteus maximus, gluteus medius (posterior fibers), adductor magnus, longus, and brevis, gracilis, pectineus, tensor fasciae latae
Joint 6	Knee	Extension	Rectus femoris, vastus lateralis, medialis, and intermedius

CROCODILE POSE: MAKRASANA

- Lie face-down with your forehead on the floor. Lengthen your legs away from you and straighten them.
- Bring your arms forward and place your hands on either side of your ears. Do not rest your hands on the back of your head, as you may add undue weight and tension to your neck.
- Draw your navel in toward your spine.

- Inhale, then lift your upper and lower body up from the floor. Keep your gaze on the floor, keeping the back of your neck long and your chin tucked in.
- Keep your legs hip-width apart, with your toes pointing away from you.
- Lift your elbows upward and keep your shoulder blades moving down the back and away from your ears and neck.
- Gradually build up to holding the pose for four minutes. Maintain an even, diaphragmatic breath throughout.

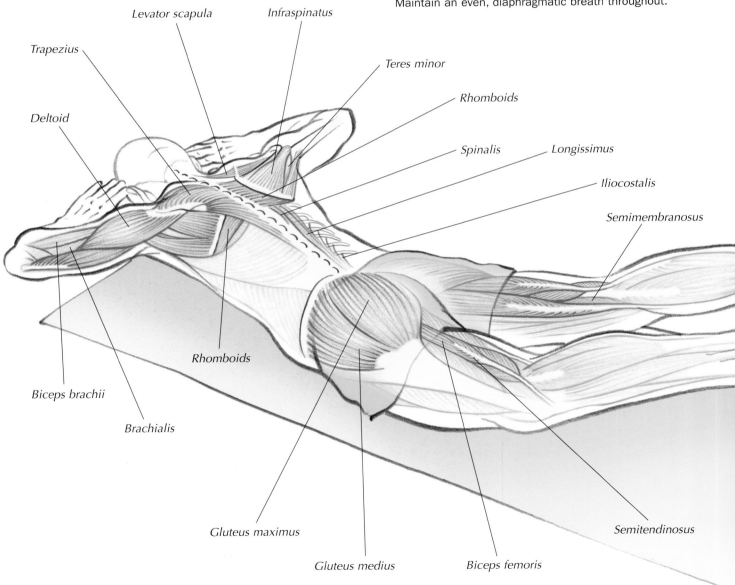

Benefits

· Strengthens both the upper and lower back muscles. Effective in increasing strength to draw the shoulders back, and in improving postural imbalances. Can help poor digestion.

Modification

· Keeping your legs on the floor will make this posture easier. To fine-tune the asana, just work on lifting your arms. Keep your forehead, torso, and legs on the floor.

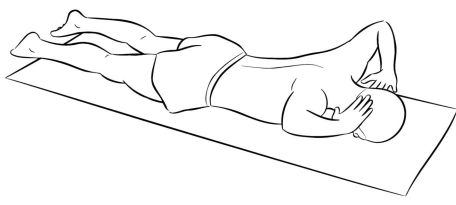

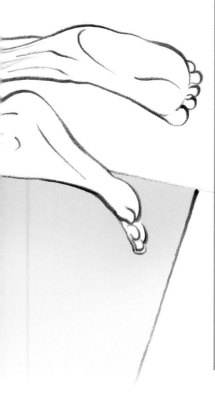

ANALYSIS OF MOVEMENT	JOINTS	JOINT MOVEMENT	MUSCLES ACTIVE
Joint 1	Scapula	Upward rotation, elevation, adduction	Trapezius, rhomboid major and minor, levator scapula
Joint 2	Shoulder	Horizontal abduction, external rotation	Deltoid (posterior fibers), teres minor, infraspinatus
Joint 3	Elbow	Flexion, pronation	Biceps brachii, brachialis, brachioradialis, flexor carpi radialis, palmaris longus, pronator teres, pronator quadratus
Joint 4	Spine	Extension	Spinalis, longissimus, ilicostalis, multifidi, rotatores, semispinalis capitis, intertransversarii, interspinalis
Joint 5	Hip	Extension, internal rotation, adduction	Biceps femoris, semitendinosus, semimembranosus, gluteus maximus, gluteus medius (posterior fibers), adductor magnus, longus, and brevis, gracilis, pectineus, tensor fasciae latae
Joint 6	Knee	Extension	Rectus femoris, vastus lateralis, medialis, and intermedius

UPWARD-FACING SPREAD-FOOT POSE: URDHVA PRASARITA PADASANA

- Begin by lying on the floor, arms by your sides, with your palms down.
- Pull your navel to your spine.
- Exhale, then bend your knees to your chest, locking the inner length of your legs together.
- Inhale, then fully extend your legs, with your heels pointing upward.
- Exhale, then press the small of your back into the floor by drawing the abdominal muscles in toward the spine.
- Stay in this pose for two or three breaths. On your next exhalation, lift your head and shoulders up from the floor, lifting your arms so that your hands are on either side of your thighs.
- Keep your tongue placed on the roof of your mouth to assist with neck stability.
- Gradually build up to holding the pose for two minutes, maintaining a diaphragmatic breath throughout.

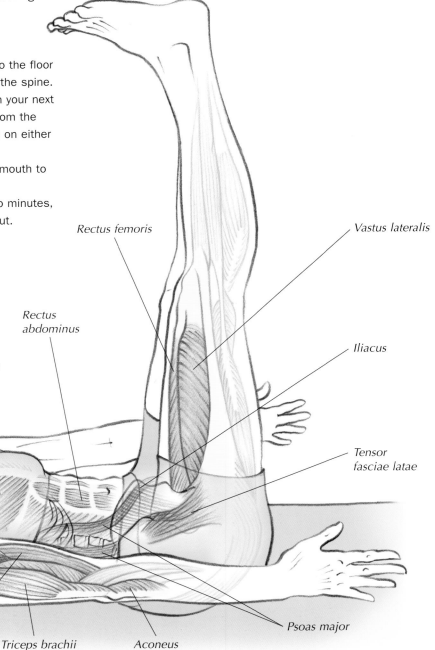

Rectus femoris

Vastus lateralis

Sternocleidomastoid

Rectus abdominus

Pectoralis major

Iliacus

Tensor fasciae latae

Deltoid

Psoas major

Biceps brachii

Triceps brachii

Aconeus

Benefits

· Improves strength in the abdominal region and teaches correct activation of leg musculature for standing poses.

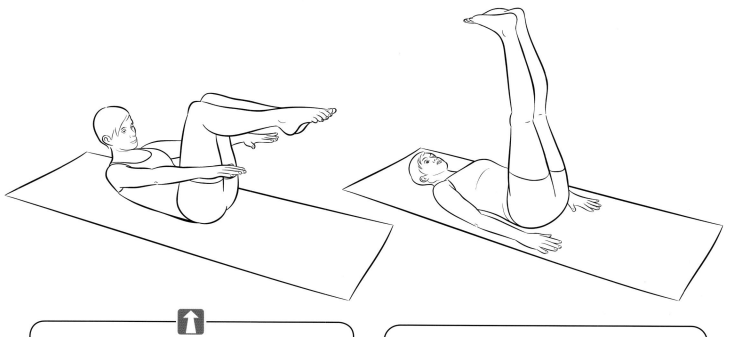

Modification

· If the full pose is too difficult for you to manage safely, keep your knees bent and gradually work up to the full asana.

Note:

· The hamstrings will stretch within this asana if they are tight.

ANALYSIS OF MOVEMENT	JOINTS	JOINT MOVEMENT	MUSCLES ACTIVE
Joint 1	Scapula	Upward rotation, abduction	Trapezius (upper and lower fibers), serratus anterior, pectoralis minor
Joint 2	Shoulder	Flexion, internal rotation, horizontal adduction	Deltoid, pectoralis major (upper fibers), biceps brachii, coracobrachalis, teres major, subscapularis, latissimus dorsi
Joint 3	Elbow	Extension, supination	Triceps brachii, aconeus, biceps brachii, supinator
Joint 4	Neck	Flexion	Sternocleidomastoid, anterior scalene, longus capitis, longus coli
Joint 5	Spine	Flexion	Rectus tbdominus, Transverse abdominus, external and internal obliques
Joint 6	Hip	Flexion, adduction, internal rotation	Rectus femoris, gluteus medius (anterior fibers), gluteus minimus, tensor fasciae latae, sartorius, psoas major, iliacus, adductor magnus, longus, and brevis, gracilis, pectineus, gluteus maximus (lower fibers)
Joint 7	Knee	Extension	Rectus femoris, vastus lateralis, medialis, and intermedius

CORPSE POSE: SAVASANA

"Sava" means corpse; this is a deep relaxation pose in which the body is motionless, appearing like a corpse. We spend most of our daily lives moving, not enjoying stillness—this is the time to experience deep stillness and inner calm.

Concentrate your mind on the subtle movements of your breath and the rise and fall of your abdomen. On each exhalation, have a sense of letting go of tension. Allow your body to surrender to gravity and try not to get caught up in unnecessary thoughts. Just allow your body to be.

· Start on your back with your heels toward the sitting bones, then gently straighten one leg at a time. Stretch your legs away from you and draw your pubic bone toward you for a second, lengthening your lower back, then relax.
· Have the legs a little wider than hip-width apart. Straighten your arms away from your body, palms up, and relax your shoulders away from your ears. Stretch your head away from your shoulders.
· Soften the skin of your face and let your jaw slightly part. Remain in the pose for between five and ten minutes.

· When you have finished, roll onto your right side. Rest here for a few moments and open your eyes. Gently bring yourself into a sitting position, becoming aware of your surroundings.
· If you find tension developing in your neck, place a small blanket underneath your neck to help keep it lengthened. You may also place a blanket underneath your knees to take any stress out of your lower back. An eyemask can be used on the eyes, as this is effective in calming the nervous system.

Benefits
· "Lying upon one's back on the ground at full length like a corpse removes fatigue caused by the other asana and induces calmness of mind" (S. Muktibodhananda, *Hatha Yoga Pradipika*). This posture gives the body time to relax and enjoy stillness and has a calming effect on the nervous system.

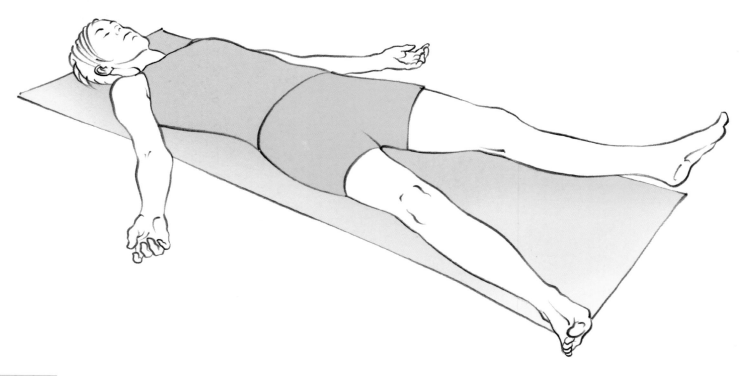

BREATHING PRACTICE

It is common with a sway-back posture for the chest to be collapsed, with the shoulders forward and sunk slightly. This position of the upper spine can coincide with collapsed breathing. This is when the optimal movement of the breath is reversed, so that, on inhalation, the chest expands first rather than the abdomen. In this pattern of breath, the belly remains soft and relatively static as the chest and shoulders lift. The breath itself is short and listless. Diaphragmatic breathing can help draw the breath out of the chest and shoulders and into the lower rib cage and abdomen, consequently stretching the intercostals and strengthening the diaphragm.

Diaphragmatic breathing

Lie on your back with your arms by your sides and your palms up. Straighten your legs, making them slightly wider than hip-width apart. Take a moment to completely relax. Try to clear your mind of unnecessary thoughts by focusing your awareness on your breathing pattern. This is the time to honor your breath and its life-giving qualities. Become aware of the quality of your breath: is it fast or slow, smooth or uneven? Once you have witnessed your breath, try not to make a judgment as to whether it is right or wrong—just acknowledge its movement and feeling.

After a few moments, wrap your hands around the bottom of your rib cage just below your chest, with your fingertips almost touching. Rest your elbows down on the floor and soften your neck, face, and shoulders. Start to direct your breath to the lower part of your rib cage and upper abdomen. As you inhale, expand your rib cage into your hands, broadening the side of your ribs. Your abdomen will lift, and your fingertips and hands will move away from each other, increasing the space between your fingertips. As you begin your exhalation, your rib cage will narrow and your hands and fingertips will move closer together. At this point, the upper chest should be relatively still, your shoulders should be melting into the floor with no tension, and your neck and jaw should remain passive and relaxed. The movement of the rib cage should be natural and smooth; try not to lift the ribs mechanically, as this will create tension and anxiety. When you first start diaphragmatic breathing, there may not be a great deal of movement; this will change over time as you start to stretch the intercostal muscles. Although your attention is on your hands at the front of your rib cage at this point, the breath will also be moving the back of the lower rib cage, increasing and decreasing the circumference of the rib-cage cavity.

Continue with this breathing for at least five minutes. Toward the end of the practice, rest your arms on the floor and see if you can maintain the movement of the diaphragmatic breathing without the guidance of your hands.

Once you are comfortable with the diaphragmatic breathing practice, progress into a sitting position and repeat the practice. You can start by placing your hands on your rib cage, but eventually your hands will rest on your knees. It is important to choose a sitting position that will allow you to maintain an erect spine.

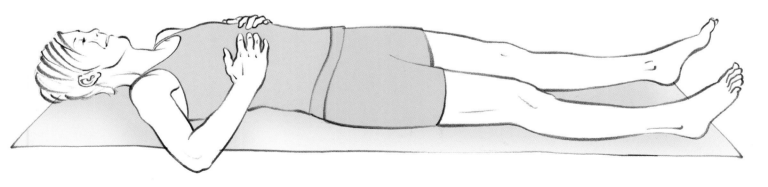

MINDFULNESS OF BREATHING MEDITATION

Many of us at some point or another have found ourselves in deep thought about some activity we should be doing or how we're feeling when we are supposed to be listening to a conversation or perhaps a college lecture. Not many people can give their undivided attention to a person or situation—we're always thinking about our next action or, when listening to a friend, relating their topic of conversation to our own experiences and how it makes us feel. We then get lost in thoughts of our past experiences when we are supposed to be focused on the conversation at hand.

Mindfulness practices are about becoming "present," about learning to become aware of our surroundings and actions with our full attention. The more we can practice the art of mindfulness through meditation, the more we will be able to carry it into our daily lives.

The method of this practice is to "tag" one number to each breath, whether it's an inhalation or an exhalation, using the numbers one to ten. This may sound like an extremely easy practice, but more often than not you will find your mind becoming distracted, and before you know it, you will have forgotten what number you were on. This is all part of the art of learning to stay present and concentrate on one point. If you do find yourself becoming distracted, gently nudge the mind back to focus on your breathing. Accept lovingly that your mind wandered off but always come back to the task at hand.

The practice

Settle yourself into a comfortable sitting position. Close your eyes and place your hands on your knees in jhana mudra (thumb and index finger together with the palms up for awareness and alertness).

Relax the skin of your scalp and forehead, soften your jaw, and allow your tongue to rest softly on the roof of your mouth. Lengthen the back of your neck by slightly dropping your chin and moving it back toward your throat. Let your shoulders melt toward the floor. Keep your spine erect and lengthened.

Once you feel your body relaxing and your mind settling, start to move your awareness to your breath.

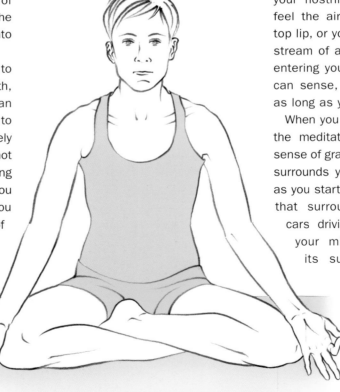

Monitor its length and quality. Try not to change your breathing, just become an observer, and pause for a few moments as you do this. Then, after your next exhalation leaves your body, mark it with a mental count of "one". Mentally count "two" after the next exhalation and continue to count consecutively to ten. Once you have reached ten, return to one again and continue for four to five minutes. Then move your focus to counting each breath just before it enters the body, again counting consecutively to ten. Repeat this for four to five minutes.

Now stop counting altogether and just observe your breath: its subtle movements in your body and its sound. After a short time, become aware of where your breath enters your nostrils and leaves—you may feel the air moving, caressing your top lip, or you may have a vision of a stream of air like a whisp of smoke entering your nostrils. Whatever you can sense, stay with that focus for as long as you can.

When you are ready to come out of the meditation, start to cultivate a sense of gratitude and love for all that surrounds you. Maintain that feeling as you start to awaken to the sounds that surround you—birds singing, cars driving past—just listen. As your mind becomes aware of its surroundings, allow your body to stretch. Gently open your eyes and try not to jump up right away. Take your time to move back into the world with a sense of presence.

REFERENCES

- Bogduk, N., *Clinical Anatomy of the Lumbar Spine and Sacrum*, Churchill Livingstone (1997)
- Chek, P., *Golf Biomechanics Certification Course Manual*, CHEK Institute (1999)
- Chek, P., *Golf Biomechanics Manual*, CHEK Institute Publication (1999)
- Chek, P., "Posture and Craniofacial Pain," chapter in *Chiropractic Approach to Head Pain*, Wilkins & Williams (1994)
- Dychtwald, K., *Bodymind*, Tarcher Penguin Group (1997)
- Gracovetsky, S., *Collagen and the Second Law of Thermodynamics*, presentation at the International CHEK Conference, London, England (2008)
- Johari, H., *Chakras—Energy Center of Transformation*, Destiny Books (2000)
- Keleman, S., *Emotional Anatomy*, Center Press Berkley (1985)
- Kendall, F. et al, *Muscles: Testing and Function*, Williams & Wilkins (1993)
- Marieb, E., *Human Anatomy and Physiology*, The Benjamin Cummings Publishing Company (1992)
- Muktibodhananda, S., *Hatha Yoga Pradipika*, Bihar School of Yoga (1999)
- Schiffmann, E., *Yoga: The Spirit and Practice of Moving into Stillness*, Simon & Schuster (1997)

FURTHER READING

- Coulter, H., *Anatomy of Hatha Yoga*, Honesdale (2001)
- Farhi D., *The Breathing Book*, Henry Holt and Company (1996)
- Kendall, F. et al, *Muscles: Testing and Function*, Williams & Wilkins (1993)
- Rosen, R., *Pranayama Beyond the Fundamentals*, Shambhala Publications (2006)
- Rosen, R., *The Yoga of Breath*, Shambhala Publications Inc. (2002)
- Saraswati, S., *Meditations from the Tantras*, Bihar School of Yoga (1983)
- Simpson, L., *The Book of Chakra Healing*, Gaia Books Limited (1999)

Nicky's acknowledgments and dedication

I would like to thank my long-term partner Richard, who has supported me throughout the writing of this book (I promise not to be a bore anymore). My mother, for her words of encouragement and love, and my father, who, although is not in this physical world, has blessed me with his spiritual presence and support throughout. To my teachers, who continue to inspire me on the path of yoga, Clive Sheridan and Shiva Rea, Godfrey Devereux and Paul Chek. Thank you to all of my students and clients who have been a constant inspiration: their love and enthusiasm overwhelms me daily. Lastly, thank you, Ann, for your words of wisdom.

Leigh's acknowledgments and dedication

I would like to thank Paul Chek, who has been the greatest influence on my career. Paul has been an inspiration, a teacher, a mentor, and a great friend. I would also like to thank my parents, who have supported me throughout my career. Without their support, I would not be where I am today. Thanks to Ross and Sarah at New Holland for their belief in my work and their support throughout the project. Finally, I would like to thank Nicky for agreeing to write this book with me—I hope I didn't drive you too crazy in the process.

GLOSSARY

Active closure is the stabilization of a joint created by myofascial (muscle and fascia) action. Often referred to in the stabilization of the sacro-iliac joint.

Afferent nerves carry nerve impulses from receptors or sense organs toward the central nervous system. Also known as sensory nerves.

Atlas subluxation a misalignment of the first cervical vertebra. Atlas subluxation can cause a disruption to the nervous system and posture throughout the body.

Compound exercise is a movement that involves a number of joints.

Contralateral refers to the opposite side.

Efferent nerves carry nerve impulses away from the central nervous system to muscles and glands. Also known as motor nerves.

Force closure is the stabilization of a joint created by myofascial (muscle and fascia) action. Often referred to in the stabilization of the sacro-iliac joint.

Form closure is the stabilization of a joint created by articular components. Often referred to in the stabilization of the sacro-iliac joint.

Hypertrophy is the increase in tissue size, often referred to as the increase of muscle tissue.

Intensity is a measure of the load of an exercise relative to the current level of strength, often measured as a percentage of one repetition maximum (1 RM).

Ipsilateral refers to the same side.

Isolation exercise is a movement that involves one joint.

Muscle spindles are sensory receptors along the length of a muscle that detect changes in the length of that muscle. Muscle spindles feed information back to the central nervous system.

Neural drive refers to the number and amplitude of nerve impulses received by a muscle.

Neutral spine is the natural position of the spine when standing without any muscle imbalances and is achieved when the cervical, thoracic, and lumbar spinal curvatures each have an angle of 30–35 degrees.

Passive closure is the stabilization of a joint created by articular components. Often referred to in the stabilization of the sacro-iliac joint—their main role.

Phasic muscles create movement across as well as the gross stabilization of joints. They have a predominance of fast-twitch muscle fibers, can create high levels of force, are quick to tire, and tend to lengthen and weaken under faulty loading.

Reciprocal inhibition is a relaxation of a muscle on one side of a joint to accommodate a shortening of its antagonistic muscle.

Synergistic dominance takes place when a synergist muscle takes over the role of an inhibited prime mover muscle.

Tonic muscles create segmental stabilization of the joints. They have a predominance of slow-twitch muscle fibers, create low levels of force, are slow to fatigue, and tend to shorten and tighten under faulty loading.

Torsion is a rotational stress applied to an object. Often referred to in the rotational force (torque) placed on the spine.

Training volume is the combination of repetitions multiplied by the number of sets and weight (intensity) used over a period of time (workout, week, month).

Type-I muscle fibers produce relatively low levels of force, contract slowly, are slow to fatigue, have a high number of mitochondria and myoglobin, and appear red in color.

Type-IIA muscle fibers contract relatively quickly and have a greater aerobic capacity than type-IIB fibers and take longer to fatigue. They have more mitochondria and myoglobin than type-IIB fibers. They favor the lactate energy pathway, have a medium-size diameter, and less propensity to muscular growth than type IIB, but more so than type I.

Type-IIB muscle fibers produce high force quickly, are quick to fatigue, have a low number of mitochondria and myoglobin, and appear white in color. These are increasingly becoming known as type-IIX fibers.

INDEX

Page numbers in bold refer to the glossary

A

More Anatomy for Strength and Fitness

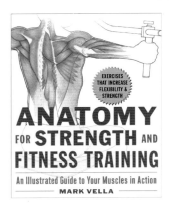

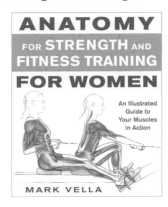

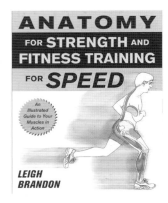

Anatomy for Strength and
Fitness Training
0-07-147533-8

Anatomy for Strength and
Fitness Training for Women
0-07-149572-X

Anatomy for Strength and
Fitness Training for Speed
0-07-163363-4

First McGraw-Hill edition, 2010

10 9 8 7 6 5 4 3 2 1

ISBN   978-0-07-163362-8
MHID   0-07-163362-6

The advice presented within this book requires a knowledge of proper exercise form and
a base level of strength fitness. Although exercise is very beneficial, the potential for
injury does exist, especially if the trainee is not in good physical condition. Always
consult with your physician before beginning any program of progressive weight training
or exercise. If you feel any strain or pain when you are exercising, stop immediately and
consult your physician. As all systems of weight training involve a systematic
progression of muscular overload, a proper warm-up of muscles, tendons, ligaments,
and joints is recommended at the beginning of every workout.

This book does not constitute medical advice. The author and publishers have made
every effort to ensure that all information given in this book is accurate, but they cannot
accept liability for any resulting injury or loss or damage to either property or person,
whether direct or consequential and howsoever arising.

McGraw-Hill books are available at special quantity discounts to use as premiums and
sales promotions, or for use in corporate training programs. To contact a representative
please e-mail us at bulksales@mcgraw-hill.com.

Reproduction by Pica Digital Pte Ltd, Singapore
Printed and bound by Tien Wah Press, Singapore